QUICK MEDITATION GUIDE

This Book includes:

Meditation Techniques

Meditation for beginners

Elliot Wood

DEEP MEDITATION TECHNIQUES

T 45 MEDITATION THNIQUS T RLIV STRSS, ANXIETY AND DRSSIN AND RETURN

TO A STATE HAPPINESS.

Elliot Wood

Table of Contents

Chapter 1

Meditation Techniques As The Secret to Live a Healthy Life

Chapter 2

Meditation Techniques And Their Benefits

Chapter 3

Top 45 Meditation Techniques To Relieve Stress, Anxiety And Depression And
Return To A State Happiness.

Technique 1 - Deep-Breathing Meditation
Technique 2 - White-Light Meditation
Technique 3 - Affirmation Meditation
Technique 4 - Walking Meditation
Technique 5 - Trataka Meditation
Technique 6 - Mantra Meditation
Technique 7 - Chakra Meditation
Technique 8 - Vipassana Meditation
Technique 9 -Raja Meditation
Technique 10 –Self-Talk Meditation
Technique 11 –Mindfulness Meditation
Technique 12 – Focused Meditation
Technique 13 – The Basic Meditation
Technique 14 - Activity-Oriented Meditation
Technique 15 - Fundamental Meditation
Technique 16 - Concentrative Meditation
Technique 17 - Zen-based Meditation
Technique 18 - Guided Meditation
Technique 19 - Yoga Meditation
Technique 20 - Traditional meditation
Technique 21 -. Binaural beats meditation

Technique 22 - Visualization Meditation
Technique 23 - Burning Flame Meditation
Technique 24 - Open Eye Meditation
Technique 25 - Zazen Meditation
Technique 26 - Point source meditation
Technique 27 - Wandering meditation
Technique 28 - Void meditation
Technique 29 - Action meditation
Technique 30 - Mirror gazing
Technique 31 - Prayer meditation
Technique 32 - Candle meditation
Technique 33 - Kundalini meditation
Technique 34 - Reiki meditation
Technique 35 - Pyramid meditation
Technique 36 - Qigong meditation
Technique 37 - Single Object Meditation
Technique 38 - Dynamic Meditation.
Technique 39 - classic sitting meditation
Technique 40 – Sweeping House Meditation
Technique 41 - Brainwave Meditation
Technique 42 - Acem Meditation
Technique 43 - Anapana Technique
Technique 44 - Body Scan Meditation
Technique 45 - The yellow light meditation

Chapter 4

Meditation Techniques And Hatha Yoga Benefits

Chapter 5

How To Improve Concentration With Meditation Techniques

Chapter 6

How To Finding the Right Meditation Techniques For Beginners

Chapter 7

How To Put Relaxation Meditation Techniques To Work

Chapter 8

The Benefits of Meditation Techniques From a Meditation CD

Chapter 9

Using Yoga to Enhance Traditional Sitting Meditation

Chapter 10

Best Meditation Technique For Beginners

Chapter 11

Tips for Choosing The Right Meditation Techniques

Conclusion

INTRODUCTION

I want to thank you and congratulate you for Downloading the book, " ***DEEP MEDITATION TECHNIQUES:*** *TOP 45 MEDITATION TECHNIQUES TO RELIEVE STRESS, ANXIETY AND DEPRESSION AND RETURN TO A STATE OF HAPPINESS*

Whenever the talk of meditation starts, the fundamental question that arises is the usefulness and effectiveness of various meditation techniques.

If you see various spiritual traditions, you will find that different people have used and developed different types of meditation techniques and they often considered their particular technique as superior as and more powerful than any other meditation techniques.

In fact I have seen many meditation masters who vehemently stress on using only their own technique and criticize any suggestion of alternative methods. This conflicting situation is a wrong way of learning meditation that eventually gives rise to unnecessary ego.

Meditation techniques are not the goal. They are simply the means to achieve a particular goal. A goal of attaining inner bliss - to attain a peaceful and tranquil state of mind.

Meditation techniques help us to progress towards this goal in a consistent and rapid manner. But the problem starts when we become too much attached to the technique itself and start considering it as the goal itself.

When you practice meditation, you must understand that in the ultimate analysis, you will have to reach a state of no-mind - a state of choice-less awareness.

The goal of all meditation techniques is to help you reach that state. Now it entirely depends upon you what kind of meditation techniques you adopt in your meditation practice.

A good metaphor is to consider our goal of meditation as the other side of a river which you need to cross through a boat. When you reach at the river side, you find that there are many types of boats. Some boats are made up of wood, some are of metal, some steamers and a few big ships are also there. As such you have many options to cross the river.

You can choose a small wooden boat to cross it, you can choose a medium size boat or you can choose to cross the river on big ship. As such it totally depends on you what kind of boat you choose to cross the river.

Their size may be different, there speed may be different, there inner comfort may be different- but all in all - they all are means to cross the river. Their purpose is to take you from this side of the river to other side. That's all.

In fact some of you may choose to cross the river by swimming instead of using a boat. That is perfectly OK as long as you reach your goal - which is to reach other side of the river.

Meditation techniques are just like these boats and ships. You can choose any of them for your meditation practice. But their final goal will be the same - to take you to a truly meditative state of mind.

They are simply the means not the goal itself. Just like a swimmer, you can create your own technique. But that will also be just a means to achieve inner bliss - not the inner bliss itself.

In this GUIDE is a comprehensive outline of 45 popular meditation techniques to relieve stress, anxiety and depression and return to a state happiness.

I hope that this GUIDE will give you enough information to point you in the direction of the meditation technique you would like to explore more.

Thanks again for downloading this book, I hope you enjoy it!

CHAPTER 1

Meditation Techniques As The Secret to Live a Healthy Life

Meditation is a technique invented by ancient Indian sages who practiced meditation in order to find peace. It is a very useful technique to relieve the stress of your day to day life and it has increasingly become popular all over the world; as people are often stressed out. They need ways to reduce the stress and that is why they are opting to meditation as the cure.

Meditation is still practiced widely in the monasteries in the Himalayas where Buddhist monks and lamas practice it in large scale and try to find "Moksha" which is the Buddhist concept for ultimate peace.

Due to the large number of people adopting meditation techniques to relieve themselves from the stress of their regular routine work, find inner peace and beauty and have the sense of freedom - even some cities have tried to replicate the environment of the monasteries and they offer yoga practices and meditation practices to people. By practicing meditation, people from all age groups have benefited largely in their daily lives.

The impact of inner peace, which is a gift given by meditation, has been observed to affect the daily life of the people practicing it and they have grown more sober and serene than before. The meditation is a minor part of the rich heritage of knowledge that is contained in the Vedas where these techniques are written in a systematic form.

Along the inner peace, every person is given a unique word which acts as the carrier of the peace inside the body of the person practicing meditation. In order to reap most out of meditation, it is very important to perform meditation in a systematic way and as per the rules as written in the Vedas.

Thus it is very important to be aware of the right meditation techniques as even though doing it the wrong way doesn't have any negative impact, doing the right way can give you more profit in terms of inner peace and beauty. Therefore it is unwise to practice it other way and reap lesser benefits from the technique.

Usually the best time to practice meditation is morning when the air is fresher than any other time of the day, but meditations are equally beneficial when performed with a calm quiet and peaceful environment away from noises and clean air at any time of day.

It should be performed in a fairly sound proof and air conditioned room of your apartment any time of the day, given that the same time is maintained for everyday practice.

In this fast moving world, mental peace is one of the biggest issues. As time is running by, we are getting more and more indulged in the busiest spheres of life. It's almost a mammoth task when it comes to extracting peace from the daily hassles of life.

Be they professional or domestic, human beings are compelled to devote a big part of their daily living to some unavoidable responsibilities and they hardly find time to analyze themselves. A deep slumber is not always the only way-out.

Meditation, in fact, can be a splendid way to remain miles from anxieties. It must be executed in a certain manner to obtain accurate results. Diverse meditation techniques are available and each of them must be executed perfectly.

With the help of several meditation techniques, you will be able to transform your dull gloomy thoughts to new and positive ones. There are certain chronological steps for meditation. Patience and concentration are the key features of meditation.

New practisers need to keep this in mind because they can never focus and concentrate until they achieve patience. Regular meditation can help you to sense your own self and can even nurture your sensory organs.

Opting for meditation techniques is undoubtedly a superb healing process that will rid your anxiety to a good extent. Owing to our hectic schedules, we often fail to free ourselves from tensions and consequently end up with certain related health problems.

Therefore, some take energizing pills to boost up for the next day. Although these artificial pills come with side effects and faster results, it's better to go for natural strategies that can in fact sharpen your intellectual powers and gear up your creativity. If you are looking for some unique meditation techniques, get them through websites. You can even download videos where instructors instruct with ample yoga versions.

A spot of absolute seclusion is a must for meditation. It should be absolutely devoid of distractions. Keep in mind, meditation is not a typical exercise that can be performed anywhere and any place you wish.

A shady tree often works fine for meditation. But it's always better to go for indoors rather than outdoors. Choose your living room where you can easily concentrate for hours.

CHAPTER 2

Meditation Techniques And Their Benefits

The benefits that people are getting are making meditation more and more popular every day. Some companies are even setting aside time for their employees to meditate, in order to be more relaxed and productive at work.

There are many easy meditation techniques that offer phenomenal benefits to those who use them. Some of these include:

Less stress. For those people who have high stress levels, meditation is an excellent way to relax and let go of these tensions.

Improved health. There are many different mental illnesses that can be benefited by meditation; depression, anxiety, and even certain levels of bipolar disorder can be alleviated by meditation, This is especially true for people who are realizing that antidepressants don't work.

Stimulates healing. Meditation can and is being used as a natural alternative for healing the body of a number of other diseases. By focusing these techniques on certain areas of the body, it allows the body's own healing power to kick in and work effectively.

A vicious circle of disturbing thoughts clutters our mind all the time. Their persistent presence prevents our mind from being focused on a particular subject. We are hardly capable of concentrating on whatever we do for an extended period of time. Except for a few, we hardly experience the 'engrossed' state of mind.

Unnecessary and incoherent thoughts make an entry into our conscious and subconscious being. Meditation techniques are the ways to mop our mind clean and make it relaxed.

It is not that the meditation practitioners face no problems in their life but they know how to efficiently tackle them. Meditation techniques not only bring them inner peace of mind but also help them fully utilize their hidden potentials to smash whatever problem pops up on the way.

A meditative state of mind requires total concentration. For the beginner, it is very hard to detach their mind from the invading problems and worries. So it requires practice to master the techniques of meditation.

One earns no benefit by fits and starts but has to practice these techniques regularly. Followings are some simple and easy meditation techniques to experience unbelievable transformation of mind.

While practicing meditation techniques, you may need a little bit of help. An experienced guide is, of course, the best source to learn these techniques from but you can also do with many meditation CDs available in the market. These CDs are not perfect or even close substitutes to an expert master, still you can learn a lot from them.

Breath control is the most popular and vital of all the meditation techniques. As this technique can be practiced during walking, playing or working, you can put yourself through a permanent process of meditation just by having full control over the breathing mechanism. Mastering the deep breathing technique not only brings subtle changes in mind but also helps the body be fit and fine.

Mental calmness, sharp thinking ability, strong perceptive power, deep intuition and peace with inner self are the various goals of meditation. One can achieve these goals through different techniques. The types and techniques of this are several in number.

You can choose any technique to meditate. However, the experts' advice is to choose the technique that best suits your mental setup and physical being – thus ensuring comfort. Meditation techniques vary on the basis of breathing, posture, sound, vision and relaxation.

One can meditate on one's inner being by listening to soft music, lying on bed in complete rest, chanting mantras in whispers or by sitting in a particular posture.

There are widely practiced techniques that work the same way. Some techniques are associated with the process of breathing. You need to focus all your attention on the cadence of breathing while in this method.

It is through the breathing that the mind gets connected to the soul and the Supreme. You can achieve the synthesis of these three abstract entities through this meditation technique. You should choose a calm place with open ambiance and fresh air. Meditation CDs can help you accomplish the art of meditation through breathing.

Beginners find it difficult to get their mind under control. As meditation is all about focusing on and delving deep into the inner world, it is not possible without control of the mind.

CHAPTER 3

Top 45 Meditation Techniques To Relieve Stress, Anxiety And Depression And Return To A State Happiness.

In specific, meditative techniques allow you to achieve an awareness of self. They do this because meditation techniques focus the mind to get past the clutter of thoughts and jumbled thinking patterns. The idea is to be able to think clearer and become more relaxed. Hence, all these techniques allow us to accomplish this.

The stresses of life can have a dramatic effect on us. As we attempt to deal with all the various problems that come our way, we are mentally worn down. Much in the same way our bodies need proper exercise to remain healthy, so do our minds need proper stimulation to stay efficient.

By becoming better attuned to our consciousness, we achieve this. In fact, practicing meditation techniques is really the only way to permanently accomplish this endeavor. If you meditate properly, you free your mind of burdensome and chaotic thought patterns. Who doesn't want to be less stressed and more focused?

Ok, so basically these techniques will help you become more relaxed, think clearer, concentrate better and more. But these things in and of themselves are not the act of meditating.

Concentrating on something is not meditation. Finding one self in a relaxing position or performing certain poses is not it either. There are a number of meditation techniques that will help a person achieve plenty of benefits in their life.

There are many other techniques that are available. These three just happen to be the most well-known and practiced in the west. What you will notice is that all three have the same goal in mind - which is to attain a higher state of awareness.

Remember, one of the most common purposes of meditating is to become better aware of the self, which in turn, produces a healthier mind. It's interesting that regardless of the differences between meditation techniques, the goal remains the same.

All of the differences in the techniques mentioned in this chapter are actually examples of how each of them lead to the same goal- that of achieving awareness. It's like the saying goes "all roads lead to Rome."

In this case, all these different techniques lead to enlightenment and awareness in addition to many other kinds of mental, psychological, social, and physical benefits. Whether the meditation technique you use focuses on sitting, walking, laying down, breathing, repeating a mantra, or chanting, it will lead to benefits in your daily life and to benefits in the lives of those around you.

Learning to meditate is one of the most important skills you can master and the sooner you learn to meditate the sooner you will gain more control over your life.

Meditation in essence is about finding your inner peace but there is more to meditation than just finding your inner peace. You can use meditation to help you in every aspect of your life. There are four core meditation techniques that every new meditator should learn.

The 45 TOP meditation techniques in this chapter cover different aspects of your life. It highlights the issue that there are varying meditation techniques you can use to improve your life. Let's look at the top 100 meditation techniques all new meditators should learn to help you in your meditation voyage.

Technique 1 - Deep-Breathing Meditation

Deep-Breath Meditation is the first technique that all new meditators will be shown. This meditation technique involves learning how to breathe and to control your breath during meditation. This technique is sometimes called the Stillness meditation technique.

Learning to use the Deep-Breath Meditation technique will teach you how to control your heart rate, your breathing and also your ability to maintain control over your mind. All of us suffer from brain-chatter where we seem to talk to ourselves.

Apart from just controlling our breathing, we start off using this technique to get control of our mind and body. Once you have mastered this technique it allows you then to use other Meditation Techniques to improve yourself. Other meditation techniques you can use are the affirmative meditation technique and walking meditation technique.

The other key advantage of mastering the deep-breathing meditation technique is that once you understand how to breath effectively using deep breaths to get control of your stress and emotions, you can use the techniques outside of meditation to quickly get control in a stressful situation. The more you practice the deep-breath meditation technique the better you will get at it.

Technique 2 - White-Light Meditation

The White-Light meditation technique is an extension of the Deep-Breath Meditation Technique in that you will use Deep-Breath Meditation to get control of your mind and body and then step into a second stage where you will use objects in your mind's eye to maintain control of your brain chatter.

Buddhist Monks have been known to teach their young monks this technique by getting them to focus on counting; however you can use any object to help you gain and maintain focus. Essentially what this technique does is to get the meditator to start by focusing on the number one as they breathe in.

Then in your mind's eye you then focus on the next number, which is the number 2 and maintain that focus as you breathe out and then breathe in again. You then change the number to number 3 as you breathe out and in again.

You continue counting through the number system until you lose control and focus. For example, if for one moment you think about the dinner you are going to have, then you must start from the number one again.

You keep following this process during each meditation session. Once you have mastered this technique you will find it is easier to get focus during a meditation session as you will not allow your mind to wander.

Technique 3 - Affirmation Meditation

Affirmation Meditation is a technique that allows the meditator to slowly train their own subconscious to follow a different attitude. For example, how many times a day to you say negative things like "That will never work" or "I will never get that job."

The objective of the Affirmation Meditation Technique is to slowly reprogram your subconscious so that you can overcome those negative attitudes with more appropriate responses. Like all meditation techniques this can sometimes take a long period to conquer but is certainly worthwhile.

Technique 4 - Walking Meditation

Walking Meditation involves learning to walk whilst meditating. I can hear it now, how are you going to close your eyes whilst walking. Well whether you realize it or not many monastic communities have regularly used walking meditation interspersed with traditional seated meditation to help break up the long periods of meditation.

The walking meditation works by getting you to first control your breathing using the Deep-Breath Meditation Technique and then to use the White-Light Meditation Technique to help learn to control your mind.

Just like I mentioned earlier with the counting technique, if you mind starts to wander whilst walking due to mind chatter, you simply stop the counting process and simply start again.

One of the other aspects you need to consider with this technique is to focus on your body and the connection your body has with its path. For each step during the walking mediation technique, you need to feel the path and each step that you are taking. For example you need to be focusing on the feeling in your feet, your ankles, your legs, your arms and so forth.

The Walking Meditation technique is one of those ones you can practice anywhere and you will probably find that it will take you some period of time to conquer this technique without your mind wandering.

Make sure that you do not punish yourself if your mind does wander or start to chatter. Simply acknowledge the wandering and bring the mind gently back into the meditated awareness and continue on your way.

Most people, when they first think about meditation, simply see it as a way to relax however your mind is an incredibly powerful tool and you can utilize meditation to change many aspects of your behavior - the way you speak and present yourself. Many professional meditation practitioners will help you to develop these techniques to improve yourself.

Technique 5 - Trataka Meditation

Trataka in Sanskrit means to look or gaze. When performing Trataka Meditation a person fixes their gaze on an external object. This can be a dot on the wall, candle flame or whatever.

Trataka Meditation is an ancient yoga practiced to develop concentration and the Ajna (third eye) chakra. Basically the person gazes at the object till the eyes begin to water.

As they are gazing they let all thoughts flow through their mind and pass away. Once the eyes begin to water the eyes are then closed. When Trataka Meditation is performed with a candle - after the eyes begin to water and are closed - the person concentrates on the image of the flame.

At first this will be an after image, but will fade into seeing the image with the mind's eye. This is a good way to develop the third eye chakra.

Technique 6 - Mantra Meditation

Mantra Meditation is where you say a word such as ohm over and over in your mind. In Mantra Meditation the word acts like a vehicle that takes you to a state of no thought. When repeating the mantra or word it is very common for the mind to drift off into other thoughts.

When this happens the person needs to gently bring their thoughts back to the mantra and start repeating it once again. In Mantra Meditation the word that is repeated is specific for the purpose of transforming the person in a spiritual way. Typically a mantra will be given to a meditator by a guru.

Technique 7 - Chakra Meditation

When performing Chakra Meditation the person will focus on a specific chakra for the purpose of cleansing or energizing that chakra. Chakra Meditation has the ability to revitalize a person's body through the cleansing, revitalizing process.

As the chakras are interrelated it is advised to start with the root chakra and work your way up when performing Chakra Meditation. When doing Chakra Meditation you can also use the aid of crystals to help in the cleansing, revitalization process. Chakra Meditation can be a powerful meditation for healing and the clearing of negative emotions.

Technique 8 - Vipassana Meditation

Vipassana Meditation is one of the oldest forms of meditation and is used for the purpose of gaining insight into ones nature and the nature of reality. The goal of Vipassana Meditation is to bring suffering to an end for the individual. This is accomplished by eliminating the three conditions which are impermanence, suffering and not-self.

After practicing Vipassana Meditation for a long period the meditator is supposed to come to a point where they separate these three conditions from themselves and achieving nirvana. It is believed that all physical and psychological conditions are not part of the true self or the "I" and should be eliminated with the practice of Vipassana Meditation.

Technique 9 -Raja Meditation

In Raja Meditation the mind is considered king and it is the minds job to tame the emotions and the body. Raja Meditation attempts to have the mind bring the body and emotions under complete control. Raja Meditation and the associated practices are a very discipline type of meditation.

When a person takes up Raja Meditation they are expected to give up things like sex, alcohol and meat and pay close attention to their actions. The idea in Raja Meditation of giving up these things is that it prepares the body and mind for meditation.

Technique 10 –Self-Talk Meditation

You are what you think. And how you talk to yourself when you are using your meditation techniques can bring you up and calm you if you know what to say. Now don't panic at the idea of talking to yourself. Self-talk is a long established meditation technique that you too can use to get your composure in the midst of your busy world.

Again, as we mentioned above, you have to let that self-talk be positive and reassuring. Remember the good of your life and your feelings when you were in control. There are other key meditation techniques that you can use that fall under the category of self-talk that can calm you and put you in a serene state of mind fairly quickly.

Remember a time when you had perfect control and try to become that person. Have a location that is always serene for you, go to that place in your mind for a moment and gather your thoughts there.

Reflect on the things in your life that give you power and self-worth. Let those things talk to you. Slowly this positive self-talk can do its magic and lift you back to a stable place and give you peace.

Technique 11 –Mindfulness Meditation

This is a meditation technique that is used by Buddhists. In Eastern origins, it's commonly referred to as "insight meditation." Mindfulness Meditation focuses on the here and now - present moment.

The goal with mindfulness meditation is to observe your thoughts. The mindfulness technique is all about focusing on what is going on around you, and more importantly, what you are feeling at the moment in time.

To start the mindful technique process you would pay close attention to your breathing, likened to the "watching breathe" technique. Focus on your long, deep and relaxed breathes until you have a comfortable and relaxing rhythm.

Then you switch to heavily focusing on what's going on in your mind. The thoughts you are experiencing and how you feel, and pay close attention to the sights and even sounds that surround you. Observing without analyzing is the key with this meditation technique. Slowly clearing your mind of any wayward thoughts and distractions.

Technique 12 – Focused Meditation

With this technique you focus on something intently but you must not think about it. You can focus on a concept, like unconditional love, or on something visual like a glass or a statue, you can focus on something auditory like the sound of the birds or waves or even on something constant like your own breathing.

Focusing on this last one is the easiest way to reach the meditation state. The concept behind meditation is simple. You have to think of yourself as a basic observer and focus on something, but just let the little narrative voice in your head do all the talking.

Technique 13 – The Basic Meditation

This one requires a comfortable position when starting and just trying to quiet your mind and think of nothing. This can be tricky if you have an untrained mind, but you'll get the grip of it eventually. The concept of this type of meditation technique is about the same as in the Focused Meditation Technique.

Technique 14 - Activity-Oriented Meditation

The third type of Meditation Techniques for Relaxation is the thinking of activities like gardening or working on a painting or practicing yoga, even walking and concentrating on the steps you are taking. It frees your mind and allows your brain to shift.

Technique 15 - Fundamental Meditation

This involves putting your mind at ease & thinking of nothing. This might seem to be complicated for those who are doing it for the first time.

A good way to begin is to stop thinking about the problems of your life and instead think of yourself as an observer of your thoughts and let them go as soon as they start materializing. The key is to witness your thoughts without putting any judgments on them.

Technique 16 - Concentrative Meditation

This is the technique which completely focuses on the concentration aspect of an individual. Either it is concentrating on the breath or an image or a mantra. It is very effective in developing the ability of an individual to concentrate, enhance awareness and free his mind from time to time mental chaos.

No specific posture needs to be maintained while following this meditation technique. Just sitting quietly in a peaceful environment and concentrating will do.

According to the yoga and meditation practitioners, an individual's breath and his state of mind are directly related to each other. Thus, concentrating on your breath will help you free your mind from troubles.

Technique 17 - Zen-based Meditation

This is the technique which is completely insight-oriented which aims at opening up the mind of people to their internal emotions, thoughts, ideas, feelings and so on. It is referred as mindfulness meditation as it enables a person know himself more.

An individual in this case sits quietly and observes everything going on around through the mind, without any need to react to any of the thoughts, memories or images.

Technique 18 - Guided Meditation

Guided meditation is currently considered the most common of all meditation techniques for beginners due to its ease and efficacy. There are various styles and methods, however the guided portion of the meditation is a reference to the guide you hear while you listen to a meditation cd.

Typically these cd's will play very relaxing music such as sounds of nature which help settle your mind to prepare you for meditation.

The guide will speak to you and set the tone of meditation as they go further in to detail describing various scenes and how to breathe accordingly. Finally, the guide will lead you into the desired meditative state whether it is sleep, goal achievement, connection to your inner self or any other reason.

Technique 19 - Yoga Meditation

Not only is yoga fantastic exercise, but it also relaxes both body and mind. Don't worry, either; you certainly don't need to be a yogi to take advantage of yoga. All you need to do is a few basic stretches, just to get your body moving in a relaxed way.

Try some very simple stretches while focusing on your breath. This will release muscle tension, create a relaxed body. A relaxed body creates a relaxed mind, and a relaxed mind promotes good sleep.

Technique 20 - Traditional meditation

Personally I wouldn't classify this as a beginners meditation technique but I've included it because a lot of people do start with this method. The idea is to have a focus point that you concentrate on, allowing your mind to get quieter as this happens.

The focus point could be a spot on a wall or ceiling. Or it could be a candle flame. Or anything else that doesn't move around too much that you can fix your attention on. A television program doesn't count for this! But a purpose made video could do - you'd watch calming pictures and listen to relaxing "new age" music.

So keep an open mind here. If you find the traditional method of meditating is too hard at first, be open to ideas that will change the method without wrecking it.

Traditional meditating can also involve repeating a mantra over and over again. One of the usual ones - you'll recognize this from Hollywood films - is the word "Om".

Which sounds a bit like a hum. Some meditation masters will pass their own mantra on to their students. The actual mantra is less important than the effect of allowing your mind to focus on the mantra and allow other thoughts and worries to fade into the background.

Technique 21 -. Binaural beats meditation

It's probably the quickest way to drop your mind into a deep meditative state that would otherwise take years of practice to achieve.

The system normally requires the use of headphones. The binaural beats are then played into your ears and your brain is placed in what can be best described as a state of mild confusion.

The two beats it's hearing are almost identical but not quite. So your mind tries to match up the two ever so slightly different tones. In the process, it gets automatically taken down to which-ever level the creator of the track was aiming for.

There are programs out there which will allow you to create your own binaural beats but unless you're a complete geek with qualifications in biology as well as computers, it's better and more reliable to buy a system off the shelf.

There are a number of different binaural beats systems available. Some require years of listening, others will get good results in a matter of weeks or months.

They'll also overlay the beats with other sound. Binaural beats on their own are a bit like listening to white noise - not exactly pleasant.

So the different meditation programs available will mask the beats with natural sounds such as rainfall or with specially designed meditation music that gives your conscious mind something to listen to whilst your subconscious mind beavers away, trying to make sense, and takes you down to a totally relaxed meditative state.

Technique 22 - Visualization Meditation

Visualization is also very powerful and it can be done by anyone, regardless of their experience. We all visualize all the time. If you don't believe me just think back to the last time you imagined anything.

That's right, you actually visualized something recently in your mind, didn't you? The difference is that while imagination can be random and can come whenever it wants, visualization is directed towards an outcome or a place you want to be in.

During your meditation you can visualize a quiet place that you can always retreat to when the stress of your days becomes too much. It will be your personal space that nobody can ever enter. Once you finish your meditation, you are again full of strength, energy and ready to tackle the day ahead.

There are so many other techniques that one would fill an entire book with them, so I will only mention them briefly here, so that you are aware that you have many interesting techniques to explore. Who said that meditation is boring?

Concentrative meditation is all about focusing on a specific object, intention or thought. Candle gazing is another interesting one. You can also gaze at a picture, at a rose, at a crystal or any other object that you like looking at.

Loving kindness is all about making you a better person, a more understanding one and it is a technique that is successfully used in healing various negative emotions.

Technique 23 - Burning Flame Meditation

The burning flame meditation is also an easy meditation technique for a beginner. Just close your eyes and imagine a bright burning candle. Really see the flame and watch it sparkle. Notice the violet, orange, and yellow colors burning brightly. Get lost in the beauty of the flame.

If your mind wanders, just bring it back to the imaginary flame in your mind's eye. This can be very relaxing. You can also do this meditation with the image of a blooming flower or with any image that you find relaxing.

Technique 24 - Open Eye Meditation

For this meditation technique, find a peaceful quiet place and something to focus on such as a flower, a fountain, or even a wall. Gaze at the object you have chosen and try to clear your mind.

Try to relax and reach a meditative state. Become one with the object you are staring at and tune everything else out. The open eye meditation only works if you are able to relax with your eyes open. Try it, to see if it works for you.

Technique 25 - Zazen Meditation

This is the technique in which you need to sit in a position symbolizing a half or a full lotus. Sitting on chair with both the hands close to each other will also do, if the first pose seems difficult to you. As soon as you get adjusted in this pose, start taking deep breaths with your eyes closed.

During this process, your mind might seem to be fluctuating from one thought to another. Let it switch, don't force it to focus on one. Within a week's time, you will find that your mind itself stops switching over to different thoughts, helping you concentrate on your breathing process.

Technique 26 - Point source meditation

This method involves focusing on a single point, single mantra, your own breath or single image. You must not allow your mind to think about anything except that point.

If you're focusing on a flame, you must reflect on the appearance of the flame and be aware of it, and avoid any unnecessary thoughts. It is effective if a person does this ten minutes every day, but for better results, you must try to increase your concentration span periodically.

Technique 27 - Wandering meditation

This method is for the abstract minded. Instead of an external source or word, simply watch the thoughts that pass through your head. The key is to not think too deeply about these thoughts or shift to memories. Do not judge these thoughts. Simply watch them.

Having a detached view of your own thoughts is a remarkably effective way to develop self-alertness.

.

Technique 28 - Void meditation

This is a rather challenging form of meditation, but once you've mastered point source meditation, it is a good idea to advance to void meditation.

Void meditation requires you to keep your mind blank- create a vast nothingness in your mind. The only thought you must have is the awareness that your mind is empty. This prominently reduces the clutter of the mind and is super effective for the anxious.

Technique 29 - Action meditation

For the fitness freaks, focusing on your body movements is also a meditation technique (this is essentially yoga!). Action meditation also includes focusing on music or beats, or any complex dynamic in your environment.

Technique 30 - Mirror gazing

Mirror gazing is one of the most simple meditations you can do. All that is involved is gazing into a mirror at your own image and reflect on how your life is going at the moment. Through these reflections, you will become more at ease. At this time you should ask the universe for whatever it is you want or desire.

Technique 31 - Prayer meditation.

Believe it or not, most prayer is actually meditation! You don't have to believe in a god or visit a church to do it either. You just close your eyes and sit peacefully, quietly and at ease giving thanks for the goodness you receive in life. Again, when you are completely at ease, this is the time you send your wishes and desires out into the universe and your subconscious.

Technique 32 - Candle meditation

Candle meditation is another very common meditation technique. There is just something so very soothing and relaxing about watching a candle flicker around back and forth. You can do it for just a few minutes or even hours.

Just focus on the flame and clear your mind of all blockages and disturbances. You will feel a massive change in state after doing so and you will feel completely at peace.

Technique 33 - Kundalini meditation

Kundalini, which in Sanskrit is traced to the word kundala (which means "coiled"), over generations came to refer to the latent power of spiritual realization buried deep down in the human body, perpetually under pressure to rise up and manifest its ultimate truths, power, and bliss. There is a relationship between Kundalini and the seven chakra energy.

Technique 34 - Reiki meditation

Reiki (pronounced ray-key) is a natural healing technique that feels like a flow of a high frequency of energy into and through a practitioner, and out the hands into another person.

Virtually anyone can learn Reiki with no prior experience or ability necessary. The attunement process opens the heart, crown and palm chakras and creates a special link between the student and the Reiki source.

Technique 35 - Pyramid meditation

Pyramid meditation may have been derived from the ancient Egyptians, they used pyramids as graves and temples but they also used them as ways to ground and convert cosmic energies.

In today's modern world, there are meditation pyramid structures that can be purchased or one can be built at home by just using pieces of wood and meditating inside.

Technique 36 - Qigong meditation

Kenneth Cohen translates Qigong as "working with life energy, learning how to control the flow and distribution of qi to improve the health and harmony of mind and body." Such practices have been prevalent in China for 2000-3000 years. The central idea in qigong practice is the control and manipulation of qi, a form of energy.

Technique 37 - Single Object Meditation

Start with something simple and not overly graphic, like a candle or a pen. Begin to gently gaze at this object and think about the object, the structure, the shape, color, size, anything that is related to the object. As you do this, feel yourself becoming physically and emotionally entangled with the object.

After a comfortable time gazing, close your eyes and see the object in your mind's eye. Hold it there for as long as you can until it begins to get fuzzy or starts to fade. Once you have determined that it has faded, or is significantly altered so that you have to imagine or recall from memory the object, open your eyes and repeat the process again.

I find that very visual people are able to do this easily and find this exercise to be fun and non-visual people have a very difficult time holding the object for even five seconds.

If you are one of those people who have a very difficult time with this, keep practicing on a regular basis and you will improve dramatically. This is a preliminary exercise and can be beneficial to practice for a few weeks before trying the other three techniques.

Technique 38 - Dynamic Meditation.

If the four stages in this simple meditation technique are followed correctly, you will have mastered a very effective meditative technique. Contrary to some beliefs, not all meditative processes involve only quiet, peaceful contemplation.

As this technique demonstrates, some forms of meditation require a more loud and energetic approach! Each of the four phases in Dynamic Meditation last for ten minutes and require a different activity. In stage one, you will prepare your body to move freely.

Breath deep and fast through your nose and move physically in any way that will increase the supply of oxygen to your lungs. For the next stage you will completely let yourself go. Dance spontaneously or even roll on the ground. Release any anger and suppressed emotions in any way you can, provided it is done safely. Screaming is recommended!

Technique 39 - classic sitting meditation

You will need to find somewhere quiet and peaceful where disturbance is unlikely. The physical position with this method can be cross legged on a pillow or, for more comfort, one can use a recliner chair.

It is not necessary to completely close your eyes, however if you do, then you should choose a well-lit area to meditate. Darkness may cause the brain's sensors to interpret the situation as time to sleep. Then the session may result in a light sleep state hypnosis, rather than a productive state of mind for meditation.

Technique 40 – Sweeping House Meditation

A wonderful, easy meditation technique is called Sweeping House! The aim of this method is to quickly clear your mind of distracting thoughts. In using this meditation technique you will place your hands behind your head then quickly brush them over the top of your head.

Use your imagination to pretend that your hands are removing all your thoughts, and with a quick flicking motion just below your forehead, sweep the thoughts away into the empty air. This can be rapidly repeated as many times as necessary.

Technique 41 - Brainwave Meditation

While it will take a bit of patience to get to the point that brain-wave meditation really works for you, in the end it is totally worth it when you begin enjoying the great rewards.

Out of all the different meditation techniques, it is only this one that brings together the science behind controlling brain-waves with the discipline of traditional meditation to provide a method that does wonders for your health and more.

This is a big reason that adding brainwave meditation to your day brings even more benefits to the time you put into meditating. It takes all the benefits of meditation, then focuses the discipline and science together so you get the very best benefits from it.

However, like other disciplines, if you do your best to be active in the process of this style of mediation, you ensure you get the most out of it that you can within the time you have to devote to it. Let's take a look at a few things you can do to get the best bene-fits from brainwave meditation.

The Process

You are probably benefiting from brainwave benefits if you have been doing meditation for some time, even though you may not even realize it. When you meditate, this is a reaction that is totally natural. Your mind is directed by you when meditating.

You put the mind into a contemplative state with discipline. Then that state is used to help provide relaxation for the body and other meditation benefits. Then, you may be able to go on to spontaneously put your body into that state, even in the middle of the day when you are working.

No matter what technique of meditation you are involved in, you are using brainwave meditation even if you aren't aware of it. At a basic level, this is a simple form of biofeedback. As you get into the program, you reduce stress with your technique of meditation, which helps to get rid of negative brainwaves.

As you go on and become more practiced, you are able to increase control and relaxation. This means you are using brainwave meditation to help accelerate brainwaves, which give you this reaction.

So, when brainwave meditation is used, you basically use the science with the process, giving yourself more tools and better knowledge. This will help you to make sure meditation is more effective and that the brainwave meditation exercises give you the best possible effects.

Technique 42 - Acem Meditation

This technique, which dates back to the 1960s, relies on the repetition of a combination of consonants and vowels that is meaningless but is believed to bring the practitioner into a meditative state.

Much research on this technique has focused on its biological benefits. But this focus does not negate the potential for this technique to help endurance runners and walkers to use it to put themselves into a more suggestible state for use with other LOA methods.

Technique 43 - Anapana Technique

This is one of the easiest yet most powerful techniques for quieting the mind, eliminating mental chatter, and cultivating deep inner peace.. Here's how to do it:

Sit Comfortably: Sit in any position that's comfortable to you. If you can sit cross legged great but if you would be more comfortable sitting in a chair, thats fine. The key is to be comfortable.

Breath naturally. Do not try to control your breathing. In this technique the breath is merely used as a point on which to fix the attention. Just breathe:)

Focus your attention. Direct your total attention on the tip of the nostrils. Be aware of the incoming and outgoing breath - on the sensation of air passing through the nostrils. Try to not let this focus waver. If it does, bring it back to your breath.

Let go. Meditation isn't the practice of stopping thoughts but merely the practice of becoming aware of them. By removing resistance and letting go of trying to control them, they fade away naturally.

Your only job here is to watch your breath with all your attention. At first, you may be faced with many thoughts and a seemingly untamable mind. But if you persist, if you simply direct your attention back to the breath every time it wavers, you can reduce the frequency and intensity of your mental chatter and begin to cultivate a calmer, more peaceful mind.

Technique 44 - Body Scan Meditation

If you're not happy concentrating on your breathing, you may feel better concentrating on your body instead; your hands and feet in particular.

So when anxiety begins...

Start off by shutting your eyes. Then, think about your left hand. Think about how it feels. What is its temperature? Does it fell comfortably warm, or even hot perhaps - or does it feel cool, or cold even? Think about what else you can discern.

If you find distractions starting to creep in, simply go back to the beginning and start again.

Continue this for a couple of minutes.

Technique 45 - The yellow light meditation

You are now going to learn the meditation called the yellow light technique. You want to visualize something you wish to come into your life and watch as you see it arriving. Get a very clear visual of this within your mind. You will see this visualization and see a glowing yellow light engulfing it.

Then slowly watch as this yellow light takes your wish or goal up into the clouds. You want to keep the vision of you receiving this in your life, now take a breath and let the light disappear far beyond your sight. Know that it is in the world gathering enough energy to manifest itself within your life.

Regularly combining yoga and any of these three techniques is a positive way of restoring health to your entire body and soul.

CHAPTER 4

Meditation Techniques And Hatha Yoga Benefits

In meditation, one practices techniques to relax, withdraw attention from the world, and concentrate on God in stillness and silence within, but many people have tensions and health problems that distract and limit them when they try to do this.

However, regular practice of traditional hatha yoga poses can relax tensions, energize your whole being and improve your health, helping you withdraw your attention from outer sensations and wandering thoughts. You practice meditation techniques to enter the inner silence.

To meditate, begin by sitting on a chair or cushion with your spine erect and your eyes closed, your hands resting, palms upturned, on your thighs. Concentrate on the breath, breathing slowly and deeply through the nose.

In cadence with your breathing, mentally say to yourself, "I am not the body" [in breath], "not even mortal mind" [out breath], "I am eternal Spirit" [in breath], "I am love divine" [out breath]. Practice this for a few minutes.

Then continue to breathe slowly and deeply with your eyes closed, but with each exhalation, sigh out the breath through your mouth making a long, drawn-out sound of "aum." This humming sound does not need to be loud. As you inhale, breathe through the nose and concentrate on the breath, and as you exhale, make the sound and concentrate on it. Feel it vibrating within.

Do this for at least five minutes; then mentally chant "aum" and, as you meditate on this sacred syllable, listen for a similar spiritual sound. Keep your eyes closed and listen with full attention. The spoken sound is an approximation of the spiritual sound. If you can hear the spiritual sound, meditate on it, and it will expand your awareness.

Gently lift your gaze with your eyes still closed and concentrate on the forehead just above the midpoint between the eyebrows. Mentally observe the flow of breath without controlling it in any way. It may slow down of its own accord if you become deeply relaxed.

As you concentrate on the breath and on the forehead with your eyes closed and turned upward, you may wish to meditate with love on a divine being or a saint, visualizing them and/or repeating their name over and over. You can also meditate on a spiritual thought or "aum." If you see divine light while gazing upward, focus on this light.

In a quiet place where you will not be disturbed, try to meditate every day, at first for at least ten minutes and as you gain self-mastery for much longer. If your mind wanders and you begin to think of material concerns or desires, keep your eyes uplifted and, as you exhale, make the humming sound and concentrate on it.

If you wish, pray or talk with God. Try to go deep. In deep silence and stillness, one may experience divine peace, love, light, wisdom and bliss. Even if you do not go as deep as you wish, meditate and seek God to the best of your ability and you will become more peaceful, more intuitive and perceptive, happier, and more aware of God's presence in your life.

Hatha Yoga

The postures of hatha yoga, the path of physical discipline, are very helpful in achieving optimal well-being. Because they dispel restlessness, tension, and fatigue, they allow the organism to right itself, to restore order and balance among its various functions.

Thus, one who learns to do the postures with concentration and breath control can enjoy deep relaxation, open up new channels of energy from within, and harmonize the functions of the involuntary organs. Better sleep and more normal blood pressure, digestion, and elimination are just a few of the physical benefits gained by practice of hatha yoga postures.

In addition, the mind is cleared of obstacles: worry, fear, inattention, complexes, frustrations, lack of self-confidence, and so on. The mind heals itself when given the opportunity, and there is no better approach to inner harmony than the practice of yoga.

Success in hatha yoga does not depend on learning to perform a great number of postures but on deepening your concentration and perfecting your technique. Practice each posture carefully, with full concentration and awareness of its inner content, and you will begin to awaken in a new way. Your mind will become clearer, your body healthier, and your spirit more peaceful.

Perform each movement slowly. If a posture causes discomfort in the head, chest, or abdomen, or pain in any part of the body, discontinue practicing it. Relax after each posture for about as long as you held the posture. This allows the heart and lungs to rest, the mind to become calm.

Set up a time to practice, in a quiet place where you can concentrate, and practice as often as you can. The muscles and ligaments must be stretched very gradually, a little more each day over a period of several weeks, and should never be forced. When your body becomes limber, you will be able to hold each posture with ease.

Individual restrictions due to age, high blood pressure, arthritis, hernia, surgery, or pregnancy should be discussed with a physician.

CHAPTER 5

How To Improve Concentration With Meditation Techniques

Concentration can be defined as the ability to focus your complete attention on a specific topic or task at hand while ignoring the surroundings and happenings around you. Focus can be classified into two categories; external and internal.

While external focus deals with the awareness that a sportsman maintains of all his team members as well as the position of his opponents, internal focus is the actual act of immersing oneself in a specific topic or activity.

The brain functions at various wavelengths, each associated with a specific brain activity; beta waves are responsible for the intense level of concentration and focus that you experience in the morning.

Fortunately, it is possible to put your brain waves in the beta frequency at will through meditation. Here is a look at some yogasanas and meditation techniques that will help you to significantly improve concentration.

1: Concentrate on your breathing: This is the most basic yet a remarkably potent meditation technique. Start in the shavasana (dead person) position or you could use the traditional position of legs crossed over each other in a sitting position with the gyan mudra assumed.

This is when your arms are extended out; palms facing upwards and you touch the tip of your index finger to the tip of your thumb, exerting gentle pressure as the other three fingers are kept straight and extended out.

Now, while in this position, make a conscious effort to expand your abdomen and chest cavity as you inhale and pull the abdominal muscles in while exhaling. Start with a deep and prolonged intake of breath and then continue breathing deeply, ensuring that you only inhale through your nose and exhale through your mouth.

This is the correct way to breathe as recommended in the yogic tradition and will help you to achieve a relaxed and calmer state of mind, as you provide more oxygen to your body while purging the carbon dioxide out of your system.

2: The shavasana position can be assumed by lying on your back, feet apart and arms at your sides with palms facing up. Close your eyes but try hard to not fall asleep. This is a deep meditation technique, so it will be incredibly relaxing and you might doze off - which should be avoided.

Now, breathe in through your nose and exhale through your mouth like in the previous exercise. However, this time you should concentrate on the sensation that you feel in your nose as the cool air enters the pulmonary system and the warm air exits out of the mouth.

3: Another way to concentrate on your breathing and achieve a heightened state of awareness and alertness which in turn will aid in improving concentration is through the use of the sound of 'aum'.

In the traditional sitting position of meditation, start by breathing in as you say aum, take a deep breath that fills your lungs with air completely continue to say 'aum' till you can no longer inhale.

While exhaling, use the word 'rheem', exhale out slowly till you run out of breath. 'Aum' and 'rheem' are both words found in ancient Sanskrit scriptures; their recitation is known to bring about total relaxation of the mind and the body and make you feel at peace and at one with the divine.

4: This meditation technique is not only very simple but can be learned in a matter of five minutes, yet it is incredibly potent in relaxing the mind and the body. Start by sitting with your spine straight, in a taut posture.

Your feet should be flat on the floor as you sit in a chair or you could fold your legs backwards with your heels and sole facing upwards and your body resting on your calf muscles.. Your arms and palms should be turned upwards and placed at the joint between your torso and your thighs.

In this exercise you endeavor to systematically relax and tense up the body to achieve superlative relaxation. Inhale sharply through the nose; go for one short inhalation followed by a long exhalation.

Now, tense your body, every muscle from your face to your toes. You should feel the energy vibrating through your skin. Hold your breath and the body position for 5 seconds before forcibly exhaling the air out of your system with one quick exhalation followed by a long slow breathing out. Feel the tension being thrown out of system with the air, repeat several times

5: While in the shavasana position, increase physical awareness of everything around you. With your eyes closed imagine moving around the room barefoot, feel the floor or the carpet on your feet, visualize every aspect of the room in precise detail as you imagine yourself taking a leisurely walk across the area exploring every nook and corner.

In the beginning, you will find it difficult to imagine things accurately, including their visual and physical feel but as your focus and concentration level increases, you will be able to see the colors of the various items distinctly and even feel their texture on your fingertips all as you lay down on the floor.

6: In the next technique, you will take long deep breaths as you try to nourish your brain and relax your body and mind with more oxygen.

This technique is known as measured breathing and should be done three to six times. Start by breathing in as you count to eight, you will need to continue the inhalation till you reach the number eight, follow this by exhaling to the count of eight.

Without pausing to take a break go into an inhalation right after the exhalation counting to eight for each. You can vary the count according to your breathing capacity. You will find that in the beginning you may only be able to reach a count of three or four.

7: You can also raise your physical awareness by imagining various sensations in different parts of your body. For instance, while in the shavasana position, try to imagine cold water dripping on your feet, or the feel of a soft rug on your soles. You will need to concentrate hard to imagine the actual feel of water or the rug.

8: A slight variation of this exercise is to sit in a comfortable position with a rose placed in a glass in front of you. Look closely at the rose, noticing every fold of the petal, the shades created due to the light and shadows.

Imagine how soft the petals will feel on your fingertips as you touch the rose while looking at it. Now, close your eyes and concentrate on visualizing the rose as you saw it.

You should be able to distinctly see every petal and even feel it on your fingertips. In the beginning, your mind will wander to the other things in the room or another thought process all together. However, you will need to teach yourself to concentrate hard on the rose. This will not only help you to calm your senses but will enhance your concentration abilities immensely.

9: Finally, trataka is another technique that works very well when used to improve concentration. Sit in a sparsely furnished room with a lighted candle placed about three feet away from you in your line of sight; that is, you should not have to tilt your head to see it. Now, look at the flame for as long as you can without blinking your eyelids.

When you can no longer hold the urge to blink, close your eyes and shift the image of the flame to the center of your forehead where your eyebrows meet, keep your eyes closed and do not open them as long as you can visualize the flame and its brightness.

In the beginning, you may not be able to go beyond a few seconds or a minute but as you practice, you will be able to continue the visualization process for twenty minutes or longer.

You will find that these techniques and yogasanas will not only help to improve your concentration but will also prove effective in helping you relax in the most stressful situations and will aid in enhancing enhance mental wellbeing.

CHAPTER 6

How To Find the Right Meditation Techniques For Beginners

Each person is apt to experience various instances of stress. No person could prevent himself from undergoing the sickening feeling of such pressure. However, various methods have been offered to aid a person in lessening stress.

One of the most frequently used ways is through meditation. However, neophytes are often troubled by fears and apprehensions on how to start developing such practice. In addition, they are uncertain about the methods and preparation they need to increase their success in this habit. This chapter will discuss the most essential meditation techniques for beginners.

The first technique to be followed in meditation is selecting the place wherein you think you'll achieve your inner peace. People have varying preferences in terms of which venues will sufficiently cater to their needs.

Make sure that you select a comfortable place, wherein you can easily organize your thoughts and achieve extreme silence. Do not meditate at public places. You should also avoid reflecting in places that remind you about stressful events that took place in the past.

Second, undergo meditation regularly. Have the drive to continue your contemplation, because it will nourish your inner soul. This means that you allot sufficient time for personal reflection. It helps whenever you remind yourself that maintaining this habit has numerous mental and emotional benefits.

Among the meditation techniques for beginners, practice the perfect breathing pattern. During this process, you have to focus your whole attention on your breath.

This will block out unwanted ideas from formulating in your brain. This may be difficult for beginners, because some ideas tend to suddenly pop in your head. However, constant practice will help you develop this skill, and as soon as you master the appropriate breathing intervals, it will be easier for you to focus on your meditation.

Fourth, try your best to not fall asleep while meditating. It would be very difficult for you to appreciate the art of meditating if you fall asleep in the middle of your contemplation.

As comfortable and quiet as your venue is, you have to keep yourself awake in order to fully grasp the happiness and lightheartedness that arise after meditation.

Fifth, learn to be patient. You cannot attain the positive results of such a form of relaxation right away. It is normal to experience difficulties at the beginning of your meditation.

However, if you learn to be patient, you will learn to develop meditation techniques for beginners that will help you in your future reflections. As time passes, it becomes easier for you to dodge mental distractions.

Meditation cannot be done by a person perfectly until and unless he knows the right way to begin it. If you really wish to start meditation and know about various meditation techniques for beginners then you should read on.

While meditating, if some kind of noise breaks your concentration then you do not need to give up. You should deal with it and try to get back to the meditative state in a short period of time. You do not need to think that once your meditation breaks, you will have to start from the start.

It is not a new thing to know that meditation poses are largely over rated. You do not need to pay more attention to difficult hand positions (referred as Mudras). Beginners need not worry about the position of their hands while they meditate. Instead, they should stay centered in meditation while maintaining comfortable poses.

It is true that meditation does not always cost a large amount of money. Over the internet, there are numerous websites which help people to learn meditation easily at a very less cost. Meditation is meant for training the mind so that it can overlook various problems and change all the negative energies into positive.

People who wish to start meditation need to understand that it will surely take time for them to learn. No one can learn meditation and reap its benefits in a very short period of time.

Patience plays a very important role for all those people who are new to the world of meditation. For beginners, there are several eBooks which offer the best meditation techniques for beginners.

If you are in search of an efficient free meditation technique, then you should know where to look for it. And the best idea is to start your search with the help of the Internet, since there are wide ranges of specialized websites that can offer you exactly what you need. This means free meditation exercises, free guidance and the techniques you need in order to relax and to reduce stress and tension.

As opposed to medications and other treatments, meditation does not come along with a package of side effects. So, basically, none of the free meditation techniques can do you any wrong. The only thing they can do is to be more or less efficient.

The answer to the above question is simple: when it comes to meditation, the only one who can observe the results is you. And if you are actually feeling better, less stressed and more joyful, then you know that you chose the right free meditation technique and that you are applying it correctly.

When looking for the best free meditation technique, you should know that the first one you read might not be the one for you. Undoubtedly, there is an impressive range of meditation exercises, from the simple ones that are destined to beginners to the most complex ones that combine numerous breathing techniques and additional equipment.

Furthermore, there are general meditation exercises that are meant to reduce stress and tension and there are certain meditation exercises that are specifically designed to ameliorate a certain health condition.

Moreover, there are meditation exercises for women, for the elderly and for other categories of people with different needs. All in all, you are dealing with an impressive range of meditation techniques, all with various roles and purposes.

Which One Is the Right Free Meditation Technique for Me?

The only one who can know the answer to the above question is you, simply because meditation works differently from one individual to another and you are the only one who will actually feelthe results.

However, when you are looking for a free meditation technique, what you should do is try several meditation exercises before you decide which one is the right one for you.

You can try both passive and active meditation exercises, you can try brainwave meditation, you can opt for a guided and free meditation technique, and you can try a candle meditation session and many more, until you find the one that brings the best range of effects.

CHAPTER 7

How To Put Relaxation Meditation Techniques To Work

I bet you can think of someone who you causes you to wonder if they have conquered relaxation meditation techniques. They seem so calm under pressure, so able to control their moods and they have such great coping skills. These are the byproducts of an effective and working relaxation meditation technique.

"Relax". That is some word isn't it? Have you had times when you "just needed to relax", but you could not? It's pretty common.

But some people know that there are ways to use relaxation meditation techniques to help them put their minds, bodies and spirits to rest. To reach that state of relaxation where they can sleep, be who they really are with friends and family or get back to work in a relaxed and settled way.

So it will pay us big time if we can get a head start on learning how to put relaxation meditation techniques to work so we have control over this important area of life as well.

Press Your Own Buttons

We all have things that relax us and things that don't. That is why meditation "gurus" work with you to select just the right focus points for you so you have objects to meditate upon that already have that power to relax you.

If anything, the daily or routine exercise of your relaxation meditation technique is a training ground for you to test out different focus points to see what brings about relaxation and what does not.

Any time you settle down for a time in meditation, you set out some goals for what you want to achieve. Part of the change of approach of designing a relaxation meditation technique is to make moving toward a higher level of relaxation a goal of the exercise.

By learning to "push your own buttons" you know precisely not only the focus points that move you most quickly toward relaxation but how to use them. You are developing your skills in relaxation meditation technique to use at other times.

Perfect Your Relaxation Meditation Technique

There is more to being able to execute a well-trained relaxation meditation technique than just using it during those times of isolation when things are calm and your environment is perfectly tuned to what you are doing.

After all, the fine-tuned ability to introduce relaxation to your mind on command is a powerful weapon in everyday life. So one of the goals of exercising and perfecting your relaxation meditation technique is to learn the key points of relaxation and how to trigger them so they become virtually "second nature" to you.

This will take time but its time worth investing in your relaxation meditation technique. As you develop your program, you will be able to reach a state of calm and relaxation more quickly. This will tell you that you are becoming an expert at your relaxation meditation technique. That expertise will serve you well when you take what you have learned and apply it in the world outside of your meditation retreat.

Take it Into Battle

Now you are ready to become like those people we talked about earlier. Except you may not be someone who was just born "cool under pressure." What you have done is that you have used your relaxation meditation techniques to train your mind in how to go to that relaxed place - even when things around you are not calm and quiet and serene.

You may find yourself applying your relaxation meditation techniques at first in calm situations where small things go wrong. A plate breaks or you get hassled in traffic. Instead of tensing up, getting angry or losing it, your relaxation meditation technique begins to take over.

Soon you are going down the well-traveled roads in your mind that you learned so well when practicing your meditative methods. You are getting the results of increased relaxation but in a real world situation.

You are getting the benefits that athletes sometimes enjoy. The benefits of your discipline are paying off in everyday life. Then as you sense your relaxation meditation techniques, finding ways to keep you relaxed under mild pressure, you can learn how to trigger those reactions when greater and greater stress comes upon you. To the world, you are a whole new person.

But you know that you are the same person, just one who has learned the discipline of staying relaxed; even when, as they say, everybody else around them is going crazy. Then people will look at you and say, "He seems so calm under pressure. She is so able to control her moods. They have such great coping skills." And at that moment, your relaxation meditation techniques have paid off to the ultimate and all your hard work will have been worth all the time you invested.

CHAPTER 8

The Benefits of Meditation Techniques From a Meditation CD

The mishmash of beliefs and misconceptions about how to meditate, what it is, how it works - and, particularly, how to know when you are doing it properly - is amazing.

As a result, many are uncertain about whether they're meditating properly, what results to expect, and how quickly these results should appear. This uncertainty leads many to quit their practice with little or no result.

The idea behind meditation is really very simple. Doing it well, however, can be difficult, and mastering it may take many years.

To learn how to meditate, you simply pay attention to a chosen point of focus - a mantra, a holy word, a prayer, the breath, or whatever - and whenever you realize you've been distracted (which can be often), you refocus.

Few scientists today dispute the benefits of meditation techniques. Respected institutions, such as the Harvard University Medical School and the Menninger Clinic, offer programs of meditation for their patients.

But many people, even with expert guidance, end up quitting; because meditation is hard to master and results come slowly.

Particularly in the first several years, the mind provides almost continuous distraction, and the meditator must continually focus and refocus the mind. This continuous need to refocus makes meditation difficult and often frustrating work, especially for Westerners who are used to instant results.

By practicing meditation techniques with a meditation CD you can help to keep things very simple. You do not have to learn how to meditate to focus your mind because the technology creates the same effect in the brain as focusing without your conscious effort. In fact, using some meditation CDs actually creates a greater effect than does traditional or even guided meditation, leading to much faster results.

With a good meditation CD, meditation is also more precise and more consistent. It does away with the preliminary mastering of a technique (which can take decades) and moves you directly to real changes in your life.

After several years of personal experience and much study I've found that that you can reach success far more quickly using meditation techniques from CDs. This is not to denigrate traditional meditation, which I practiced for many years prior to my use of meditation CDs, and for which I have great respect. But the results speak for themselves, and results are what most people are interested in.

If you're experienced with traditional meditation techniques, you will find that using a meditation CD program allows you to meditate more deeply and create much greater positive change.

And, if you've never attempted meditation because you didn't think you had the time or talent to devote to it, you may discover how easily you can fit these meditation techniques into your life.

Even guided meditation techniques can be hard to master with so many distractions throwing us off the trail. But by learning how to meditate with a meditation CD you can quickly and easily start to experience the full benefits of meditation.

CHAPTER 9

Using Yoga to Enhance Traditional Sitting Meditation

The art of yoga and meditation will de-stress your life and put your emotions back in balance. Learning new meditation techniques could open up a whole new world of possibilities for your yoga meditations.

Breathing techniques are extremely important for yoga meditation. By focusing on your breathing patterns, you will be able to break down your thoughts and empty your mind.

Visualize the passage of air passing through your mind to create a feeling of emptiness within the skull. Once all thoughts are removed from the mind, the meditator is able to explore his true Self.

Pranayama are the breathing exercises used for yoga. The art of concentration needs to be mastered, as when concentration is maintained, meditation is achieved. Aim to relax during meditation and breath smoothly with no obstructions.

Once you have attained a comfortable position to meditate, then spend about 5 minutes practicing breathing techniques. By performing humming or Aums, you can help lengthen your breathing exhalations. This will produce a calming effect on your nervous system and allow smooth, rhythmic breathing during your entire session.

Self-Illumination Meditation is one of the techniques that perhaps you would like to follow. This technique aims to expand illumination within the mind and makes use of awareness to eliminate darkness from within. It is possible to move awareness throughout the body. Prana is an energy that is purposely moved by the meditator.

By moving awareness into areas of the body that feel dark and lifeless, we are able to illuminate them and rid them of the darkness. In this meditation technique awareness will initialize from within.

Exploration of the mind and body is not done with the eyes, but with our higher conscious awareness. The beginning stages of this technique are joyful. The meditator awakens inner light and enjoys taking the time to balance it.

Raja yoga is a meditation technique where the meditator will be filled with joy or bliss. In Raja yoga a relationship with God will be established. Another technique is Zazen or Zen meditation. The objective of this technique is discipline.

In practicing this method, one will realize how much precious time can be wasted in our everyday lives. It is usually performed in the lotus position. Your back should be straight and chin tucked in. Body weight is evenly placed on both of the legs.

CHAPTER 10

Best Meditation Technique For Beginners

Meditation technique could help you in dealing with today's life that is full of struggles and stresses. If one decides to slow down, there is a full chance of being left behind.

Most of us live a stressful life and are overloaded with work to maintain pace with others. Stress is the gate to all mental and emotional ailments. Meditation is the best possible way to reduce stress and live a healthy and happy life.

Meditation traditionally is done by focusing on objects like a candle, or your breath. Through meditation, your mind and body relaxes and you experience inner peace. The more you are focused and concentrated, the better results you are going to experience.

Meditation helps in developing your concentration levels. Many people amongst us believe meditation is not for us and might not work in our situation. Well, this is completely wrong and the fact is that anyone can easily learn meditation. If you practice it regularly it will help in knowing yourself better.

The most basic form of meditation technique is closing your eyes and counting your breaths. All you have to do is to simply breathe in and breathe out and pay attention to the sensation of your breath coming in. You have to feel the air coming in and going out of your nostrils.

This will help you concentrate or meditate. When you will follow this 'breathe in and breathe out' for some time, you will notice that your focus on counting your breaths is increasing and your contact with the outside world is reducing. Keep your eyes closed during this process and keep yourself focused.

Another common meditation technique is the use of some mantras. In traditional Hindu culture, the word OM is considered magical for healing powers. The skill lies in not just speaking it but chanting it from the bottom of your heart.

It can be any mantra, all you have to do is to chant it again and again so that your mind starts focusing on it. When you chant anything repeatedly by sitting in a quiet room and closing your eyes, you will start noticing that your contact with the outside world is reducing.

Meditation technique is very similar to technology in its development. From the early stage until now, meditation has undergone a lot of changes. Now, with advanced but yet very simple technique, meditation becomes very easy to do.

One of these techniques is the initiation technique. After getting a Divine Energy initiation, you could get into a deepest meditation state instantly. Getting into deep state of meditation requires months and months of intense training in the past, but this can be achieved almost instantly with Divine Energy initiation.

If you think positive thoughts during meditation, it will have a positive effect on your body as your thoughts have a direct influence on your body. This is called self-healing meditation which is involves deep meditation.

Through this, positive energy is produced in our body that increases the healing process. This form of meditation is often suggested by hospitals these days.

For meditation, you should be in a calm and quiet place. This will help you to focus in a better way. The mattress you are practicing on should be comfortable too or else you will easily get distracted. Early morning is the best time to meditate as mind is usually fresh at that time.

Drinking a glass or two of water prior to meditating is good. One thing to keep in mind is that you should not eat too much before you start meditation. Keep yourself light and your mind relaxed. When your stomach is neither empty nor extra full, you can concentrate better. Whatever meditation technique you choose, enjoy it.

CHAPTER 11

Tips for Choosing The Right Meditation Techniques

There are so many different meditation techniques out there that the choices can often be a little overwhelming. There are simple techniques that just require you to sit in a quiet corner, thinking about nothing, which can be hard for some people to do.

There are other techniques that require you to get into physical positions that can test the limits of your body, and some people may not want to get all bent out of shape, so to speak. With so many different ones to choose from, here are some tips to help you choose the technique that will work the best for you.

The first place to really start is by thinking hard about what you want meditation to do for you. Sure, everyone wants to beat stress, and you can do this with simple relaxation techniques.

On the other hand, some people are looking for specific reasons to meditate, maybe for getting rid of some ailment, or to help themselves heal from an accident or injury. Knowing what you want to use meditation for can help you find the right one.

The next big tip is finding a technique that you are going to be able to do. Going back to techniques like Yoga, with many different positions to bend your body into, holding a pose for minutes at a time, etc.

Many people just can't or don't want to put that amount of effort into meditation, or may not even be able to hold some of these poses. It is a good idea to go online and look up some of these meditation websites and see which ones are going to be the easiest to start with.

Now this next tip is important. You don't have to pay hundreds of dollars to learn meditation. While some sites offer to teach you to meditate for a price, there are many others that offer the same information free.

There are many good techniques like specific forms of meditation and Yoga that do require some kind of money. However, these are for more experienced people. They also require a certain level of commitment, and in many cases, there are also additional costs if you want to get into deeper states of consciousness.

Another important tip for finding the right meditative techniques is to keep at it. Some people find the right form right away; others try several before they find the right one.

It can even be helpful to use a combination of techniques to help you. Some use deep breathing exercises to start out with, to help them get relaxed, them move into meditating.

Always find a technique that you can stick with. If it is too complicated or takes too long to do, then skip to another. All too often beginners have lofty expectations, start doing some complicated form and wind up giving up in frustration.

If you are really serious about learning meditation techniques to help improve your life, ease some of the tensions you may be experiencing... finding the right format can really help you achieve your goals, whatever they may be.

CONCLUSION

The term meditation is not new to the present world. In fact, it's been one of those ancient arts in maintaining your bodies mechanism. Although the concept of meditation rose with the saints, the importance of the meditation techniques came to be realized in the later part of the 20th century.

Compared to the earlier times, the new age has brought more newer and effective meditation techniques. In today's world, meditation is a must because it's impossible for the human mind and body to relax while tackling daily tensions and worries. The prevalent techniques of meditation can be divided into two categories - Concentrative meditation and Zen-based meditation.

To kick off with concentrative meditation, it focuses on the breath based on a sound mantra that helps the mind achieve relaxation and get rid of fickleness. One of the fundamentals of concentrative techniques is to sit calmly and concentrate on the working of your breath.

According to the age-old belief of the yoga practitioners, meditation introduces a direct correlation between one's breath and state of mind. For instance, if a person is agitated or frightened, his breath tends to turn shallow and uneven. On the contrary, a slow and deep breath is observed in case of a calm mind. This is one of the meditation techniques to test your mental equilibrium.

One of the vital meditation techniques for anxiety is to get into the regular habit of inhalation and exhalation. This helps to sharpen your focus and enhances your imaginative and concentration power. While you focus on your breath awareness, your mind takes up the rhythm of inhalation and exhalation.

Therefore, your breathing gradually slows and your mind gains tranquility and calmness. This is one of the most efficient meditation techniques whichs brings stunning results in your work place and lets you accomplish your work targets quite comfortably.

Zen based or mindfulness meditation is meant to focus on the sensations and perceptions passing to and fro within a human body. It's one of those meditation techniques that help to control your feelings, emotions and anger. This wonderful technique also makes you aware of images, thoughts, sounds and even smells.

Here, you simply need to sit quietly and witness everything that passes through your mind. While your brain conjures certain memories, thoughts and worries, you are not supposed to react and should instead sit calmly and observe. It is undoubtedly one of those brilliant techniques that helps you to get rid of worries and anxieties.

Yoga Nidra helps you achieve a complete detached frame of mind. These techniques for anxiety are ideal for reducing anxiety to a great extent. Yoga helps the individual to penetrate into the inner recesses of mind and concentrate harder.

Thank you again for downloading this book!

MEDITATION FOR BEGINNERS

A PRATICAL AND EASY GUIDE ON HOW TO MEDITATE

Elliot Wood

Table of Contents

Introduction

Chapter 1

What Is Meditation?

Chapter 2

Benefits Of Meditation

Chapter 3

The Biggest Obstacles to Meditation

Chapter 4

Types Of Meditation That Beginners Can Get Started With

Chapter 5

Powerful And Proven Meditations For Enlightened Living Full Of Love And Success

Chapter 6

How to Choose a Meditation

Chapter 7

Steps to Set Up For Successful Meditation

Chapter 8

Equipment For Meditation

Chapter 9

Frequently Asked Meditation Questions From Beginners

Chapter 10

Developing Your Weekly Meditation Plan

Chapter 11

Tips On Meditating For A Healthy Mind And Body

Chapter 12

My Own Meditation Journey

Conclusion

INTRODUCTION

I want to thank you and congratulate you for Downloading the book, " ***MEDITATION FOR BEGINNERS*** - *A PRACTICAL AND EASY GUIDE ON HOW TO MEDITATE*

Meditation is one of those kinds of things that you have probably heard about but you have never tried. Maybe you think it is one of those kinds of new-age type things that are all promise and very little substance, but you are genuinely curious to try it out.

Many associate meditation with the old Buddhist monk in his orange robes, or perhaps somebody secluding themselves in a far off temple for several years. Well, beginners learning to meditate will not have to retreat to a secluded temple to get hands on experience, you won't have to visit a cave or grow a beard either. All you have to do is relax.

It is no secret meditation has been considered a part of modern day medicine. It is also known that the health benefits of it can be nothing short of amazing. If you would like to enjoy a healthier lifestyle by harnessing the power of meditation the read on...

For complete beginners, Meditation could be very confusing, boring and discouraging chore to do. To the western cultures, sitting quietly without a word for a long period of time is not something you learned in school or from your parents, unless your parents are Buddhist.

More and more westerners are introduced to the great benefits of Meditation, but find it too difficult to do. Although there are a lot of scientific evidence of the benefits of Meditation published and made available now, most people know Meditation from movie or books picturing an Indian Yogi with long beard meditating naked under a big tree, spending most of his life time doing so.

Meditation is generally getting into ones inner being. Listening to the environment, the chirping of the birds, listening to ones breathing and hearing the breeze of the air is one way of meditation for beginners that cannot be compromised.

Meditation is a process that gives you a chance to discover your own inner self. Several meditation techniques are available that can be adopted by individuals easily. To know the steps that could make meditation for beginners a bit easier, following the guidelines in these chapters will surely be a great help.

Meditation for beginners can be done easily with one simple trick. Once you have discovered it, you'll quickly be able to get into a mindful meditation to relieve stress as well as having found an excellent meditation for anxiety relief. This book gives you that trick as well as more resources for starting your meditation process like a pro.

Meditation for beginners can often be a daunting task. How do I start? What should I feel? Am I doing it right? These are just some of the questions a beginner will ask him or herself when they start to learn to meditate.

The following chapters will provide some tips on how to start to meditate for beginners. These are basically the same techniques that are used by the experts. A beginner must be totally focused if he plans to make progress in this great journey.

How to meditate for beginners can best be approached with an unfolding, allowing, or quieting. The beginner doesn't need to accomplish much. The beginner wishing to start the practice of meditation must first determine to set aside the time required.

Time must be invested, but don't be concerned with "filling the time" with anything. Just allow the time. Meditation is not so effective on the run, especially in the beginning.

Meditation is one of the great eastern practices that has started to take hold in western culture. In fact, people all over the world are benefiting from it, both in mind and body.

So, why isn't everyone meditating?

It could be that not everyone knows of all the amazing benefits like increased relaxation, and decreased levels of anxiety and depression. This BEGINNERS GUIDE contains a rundown of only some of the many benefits of meditation, and a set of instructions for starting your own meditation practice.

Thanks again for downloading this book, I hope you enjoy it!

CHAPTER 1

What Is Meditation?

Meditation is the practice of focusing on an object or a single point of awareness. It is the practice of calming the mind to allow one to become immersed with their true essence; the true self that is one with all (source, universe, divine consciousness, universal consciousness or any other given name meaning the same).

As you will discover there are lots of approaches to meditation; hundreds of different tips and techniques. These all work; certainly in the beginning they help to focus your concentration. It is, however, important not to get attached to a particular technique or object.

When it comes down to it meditation is all about a post realization that you have discovered the secret gap that is as Wu describes; nothingness, emptiness, nonexistence. Only then are you meditating, and the key is not to grasp what you have discovered but, simply allow it to be, merging with the stillness, the silence and the tranquility that is the pure essence of our universe.

It is the path to all wonder and the gate to the essence of everything. It can only be found within, by merging with the silence, the stillness and the tranquility of the present moment.

It is discovering meditation and the secret gap that leads to a life of fulfillment, happiness, and total inner peace. Life becomes flowing, effortless, and beautiful and at the same time you achieve self-awareness which brings clarity, creativity and a deep sense of true purpose that is simply just being.

Meditation existed before history was recorded. Archaeologists found ancient Indian scriptures which detailed the practice of meditation dating back thousands of years. It is a well-documented practice of many world religions to include Buddhism, Christianity, Hinduism, Islam, Jainism, Judaism, Sikhism and Taoism.

Spreading from the East meditation techniques are now practiced throughout the world by millions of people on a daily basis. Meditation in Sanskrit is DhyÄna and is one of the eight limbs of yoga which leads to a state of SamÄdhi (joy, bliss or peace). The physical practice of yoga, through the avenue of the breath, is in itself a moving meditation which again is practiced by millions of people throughout the world.

Studies have shown that meditation decreases the negative effects of stress, anxiety and depression. Overall we become calmer, happier and more fulfilled. Meditation improves concentration, which is essential to realizing our true potential.

Focused concentration generates great power and when our powers of concentration are improved we are able to use this not only for the purpose of meditating but in our other activities too. Part of achieving our goals and desires is having the ability to master our thoughts.

By calming the mind and focusing our concentration, we are able to experience this self-mastery and we can begin to change and replace our negative or unwanted thoughts with positive ones.

This shift in our thought process aligns our energy with that of universal energy vibrations and we will begin to notice positive changes and improvements throughout all areas of our lives.

Physically, meditation reduces stress related symptoms such as heart palpitations, tension and migraine headaches, disturbed sleep and nightmares and hypochondria. As stress and anxieties are reduced we are actually decreasing the probability of experiencing any heart related illnesses.

Studies have also shown that meditation can relieve chronic pain, drop cholesterol levels and improve blood pressure. The flow of air to the lungs increases and improves and we will experience an overall greater sense of wellbeing.

Buddhism often describes meditation as a way of 'training the mad monkey', referring to the mind as a mad monkey, which is always jumping and racing from one thought to the next. During an average day we think around 64,000 thoughts!

The Buddha said by the absence of grasping - one is set free. Meditation is not something you achieve by trying. Although when you begin to practice you are seeking to meditate effectively, the more you try the more it will elude you. Meditation can be likened to holding a wet bar of soap; one minute you are holding it in your hands and the next it's slipped through your fingers.

Meditation is about letting go and to discover the secret gap you have to let everything go. Let go of any outcome before you begin. There are many meditation techniques, and over thousands of years different meditation practices have evolved.

The true essence of meditation, however, is just to sit and be. Quite simply you are going beyond the 'conditioned' mind and elevating your mind to a state of pure self-awareness.

Whilst you can focus on an object or on your breath to help you to reach this state, ultimately it is a natural process which evolves over time, the essence should always be in connecting yourself with your source. You are looking inward without actually attempting to do anything but to just sit and be.

It is also effective to meditate on particular struggles or problems we are experiencing in our lives. For instance, if we want to come to a decision on a particular aspect of our life; a career direction for example, meditating on this can help us to arrive at the answer.

At times the answers we are seeking can come into our minds almost immediately. The power of focusing concentration and directing that focus towards a particular question or subject can produce amazing results.

CHAPTER 2

Benefits Of Meditation

Meditation for beginners benefits not only your mind, but also your body and soul. Meditation has numerous advantages that would take a whole book to write about. Here I will mention the most important benefits and the most overlooked benefits that meditation provides.

The Most Important Benefits of Meditation

It is very useful to read about meditation benefits if you are still unsure whether you want to start meditating. These benefits will help you decide if meditation can contribute to your well-being and improve other aspects of your life.

1. Meditation improves your focus

One of the greatest meditation benefits is its ability to increase your focus. Once you start meditating, you will be able to effortlessly concentrate on any work you do without getting distracted.

That will make a huge difference in your life as you will significantly increase your productivity. You will be much more successful than the average person who cannot sit still for more than 5 minutes.

2. Meditation makes you aware of your thoughts

During meditation you will need to focus on silence. That means that you will be able to spot your thoughts as soon as they come in. This will give you an opportunity to judge your own thinking.

For example, you will be able to check if the majority of your thoughts are positive or negative.

You should not be surprised if you find the latter to be true because negative thinking is almost a default thinking for the majority of people.

3. Meditation reduces stress

Meditation almost instantly reduces stress as soon as you start practicing it. This is because during meditation your whole mind is cleansed from negative thoughts.

You can sometimes even feel the cleansing process whilst meditating. When you feel energy circling in your head, it means that the intensive cleansing process is taking place. It is a very interesting feeling, I must say:)

So when your mind becomes more pure, you will have less negative thoughts. As a result of this meditation benefit, you will not be suffering from thoughts of worry and fear.

Of course, you will not be able to get rid of all the negative thoughts you have (especially if you keep introducing new negative thoughts after meditation). However, if you constantly meditate, your main mental state will remain positive.

4. Meditation develops patience

If you meditate daily, you will remain calm and positive during the times when most people lose patience. For example, waiting in a queue will no longer be of concern to you. When you are stuck in traffic, you will feel as good as when you spend your time at home.

5. Meditation gets you into the state of joy

Another great meditation benefit is that sometimes you will become happy for no reason. Your surroundings will look magical and you will see everything in different colors. Such state of joy will usually last just for a minute or so, but with time this will increase.

Being in the state of joy means that you will see yourself as a very happy person. You will perceive your life to be without any problems. Whilst you are in the state of joy, the positive energy inside you will look for ways to express itself.

Therefore you will be able to express it anyway you wish. You may think of doing something creative, pursuing your goals or spending time doing something you really like.

6. Meditation helps you achieve inner peace

One of the meditation benefits is clearing your mind from negativity. Because of that you will become peaceful as there will be less worrisome thoughts left in you.

You will notice a huge difference once you develop inner peace. This will feel as stillness inside you. Even if someone tries to upset you or make you angry, you will not give in because you will be strong inside.

External circumstances and events will affect you less because your main concentration will be inside you, rather than outside. You may still get a bit emotional on the outer level, but deep inside you will remain still and peaceful.

7. Meditation detaches you from negative emotions

During meditation your mind is cleared from useless thoughts. As fewer negative thoughts will be left in your mind, you will experience less negative emotions. This is because all your emotions result from thoughts.

Besides that, even if you still feel negative emotions, they will not affect you greatly. This is because during meditation you will be able to observe your thinking.

Once you think about something negative, you will be aware that you had a negative thought. The thought will not have control over you as you will spot it before it could overwhelm you with some emotion.

8. Meditation makes you aware of emotional harm

This is a great meditation benefit. With the practice of meditation you will be able to feel what harm your negative emotions do to your body, mind and soul. This new awareness will make you wonder if you want to get into the negative state again and therefore you will avoid arguments and other harmful situations.

You will also become more sensitive to the energies of other people. You will sense from a distance if a person is angry, upset or happy. That will benefit you greatly because you will know which person is better to be around. By only being with positive people you will avoid being dragged down into low emotional states.

The Most Overlooked Meditation Benefits

These meditation benefits may or may not apply to you.

Meditation Benefits... It depends if you are interested in becoming more conscious and aware of the universal laws as well as higher consciousness. Even if you are not interested in the subjects above, it might be worth reading the rest of the chapter so that you would not miss out on something beneficial.

1. Meditation makes you connected with the universe

This is an amazing meditation benefit. When you practice meditation, you start feeling connected to everything in this universe. You understand not only human beings, but other forms of life, like animals. I do not mean to say that you will understand their communication methods :) However, you will be able to sense how they feel.

You will feel emotions of animals when you pay close attention to their behavior. So when an animal is scared, you will feel the fear he has. I find this ability amazing because then you can sense when animals are happy and express compassion when they feel upset.

When you start understanding how they feel, you will look at animals in a different way. You will no longer see them as some external beings that are complete strangers. You will feel connection with them at some level. And that connection is the consciousness that we all have.

Because of this meditation benefit you will understand nature better. You would not tear a leaf off a plant, for example, because you will know that plants can feel the pain.

2. Meditation raises your consciousness

Meditation naturally raises your consciousness because you start seeing the true colors of life. You see abundance of everything rather than lack, you feel that the world is going into harmony rather than getting deeper into chaos.

You start understanding the truth. Instead of relying on media for information (which is almost always depressing and false), you find all the answers in your consciousness.

3. Through meditation you connect with the universal mind

That is one of the best meditation benefits that I have found. Once you are used to meditation and you have made it into your daily practice, you will experience a flow of ideas at some times.

For example, you need to come up with some business idea and but cannot think of anything. All you should do is to ponder on that for a while asking yourself 'What are the best business ideas I can think of?'

After that just let go of this thought and meditate at normal times. You will notice soon that you start getting business ideas from different sources.

You may read a book and some words will catch your attention and you will realize that this is a great topic for your business project. Such idea may come in a form of your thought. Or some friend might introduce some idea that you can apply for your business.

The ways ideas from source can reach you are really unlimited. Just be open to receive them by being aware of what is happening around you.

4. Meditation removes obstacles for manifestations

When you visualize and try to manifest your desires, meditation practice will be of great help.

Meditation eliminates most of your negative thinking. Negative thoughts are nothing more than limited beliefs that you kept reinforcing until they became unconscious. So once you get rid of them, they will not block your desired manifestations from reaching you because there will be no external forces clashing with your positive intention.

5. Meditation raises your vibration

Meditation benefits you immensely in raising your vibration. After you finish meditating, your vibration might fall a bit, but if you practice meditation constantly, your entire vibration will be raised.

When you get into the higher vibration you become vibrational match for positive circumstances and events in your life. This is because by raising vibration you change yourself into more positive, loving, peaceful and happy person.

After a week of meditation you will start seeing and sensing first meditation benefits like reduced stress, inner peace and inner strength. When you keep meditating for longer, you will notice much more benefits including the ones that I have mentioned in this chapter.

CHAPTER 3

The Biggest Obstacles to Meditation

The sad truth is that while most of us are aware of the benefits of meditation, very few of us actually have a regular meditation practice. There are a lot of obstacles to overcome in order to incorporate meditation into our daily lives.

I overcame those obstacles and have been meditating daily for two years as well as meditating periodically throughout the day! Through meditation I have experienced more peace and joy in my life, I've become less reactive and less stressed and I have more energy and creativity! And I know you can experience these benefits as well!

Many of us have misconceptions about meditation. The most common misconception is that meditation is about getting rid of thought! That would set anyone up for failure! Meditation, rather, is about becoming the observer of thought rather than the reactor to thought.

Meditation, pure and simple, is being fully present in the moment! In this meditative state you are aware of the truth of who you are beyond your body and your mind.

Have you ever been in awe at a beautiful sunset?

So much so that you forgot about what happened 5 minutes ago, and you weren't thinking about the future? You were completely in the moment and had this sense of aliveness inside? Well, that's meditation!

So now that we know what meditation is, how do we incorporate it in to our daily lives? I knew the reasons why I had struggled for years before I developed a regular meditation practice, but I was curious to see if others had the same reasons. So I conducted an international survey on the biggest obstacles to meditation. Below are the top six biggest obstacles to meditation, and how you can overcome them!

1: Not having enough time

The biggest obstacle people face in developing a regular meditation practice is TIME. We don't have enough time to meditate! (Interestingly enough this wasn't just an "American" phenomenon.

People from all across the globe mentioned they didn't have enough time to meditate). Yet there are 4 simple ways to incorporate meditation into your life without taking ANY time out of your current schedule!

First, I invite you to convert your waiting time into meditating time.

The average person waits 45-60 minutes a day. We wait for appointments, we wait in traffic, we wait in line at the grocery store and we wait on hold on the phone. Yet those precious "waiting times" can be converted into meditating times.

So next time you are waiting for an appointment, take a moment to notice your breath. Or next time you are waiting in line at the grocery store, take a moment to smile from the inside.

Second, have a daily activity be your meditation. You can incorporate meditation into any of these daily activities:

- brushing your teeth
- emptying the dishwasher
- showering
- eating

- walking
- folding laundry, ironing

As you brush your teeth, notice your breath. Or notice the aliveness in your hands and mouth. As you empty the dishwasher, feel the aliveness in your hand as you put each dish away.

Third, have your dog or cat be your meditation! Have you ever noticed when walking your dog how your dog is completely in the moment, taking in its' surroundings? Well you can join your dog in this blissful state.

When walking the dog notice the aliveness in your feet with each step. Notice the aliveness of the trees, birds, your surroundings. While petting the cat, notice the softness of the fur. Be completely present with your dog or cat!

Four, meditate while driving! Now, of course, do NOT close your eyes and meditate while driving. But you can be completely present while driving, with your eyes open. While driving, notice the aliveness in your hands as you touch the steering wheel. Or at a stop sign or in traffic, notice your breath.

These are simple ways you can incorporate meditation into your daily life without taking ANY time out of your current schedule. If we all did these simple things, we'd have a daily meditation practice!

2: Lack of Self-Discipline

The second biggest obstacle people face in incorporating meditation into their daily life is lack of self-discipline! Meditation takes discipline. I know many of us start out with great intentions to meditate daily or to exercise daily and we might do it for a couple of weeks, but then we lack the discipline necessary to continue.

That's why life coaches, personal trainers and other professions have been created! To hold us accountable and to keep us focused. So if you lack self-discipline, find a meditation partner! Ask your spouse, partner, friend, coworker to join you in incorporating meditation into your daily life. Hold each other accountable.

Or even if you can't find someone that wants to meditate with you, tell your spouse/friend/partner/coworker of your intention to meditate daily and ask him/her to check in with you and ask you how you are doing. Just as an exercise partner is beneficial and productive, a meditation partner can be too!

3: Not having the right place or space to meditate

The third biggest obstacle people mentioned is NOT having the right place or space to meditate! This is a "perceived obstacle." You can literally meditate anywhere; while driving a car or walking through a crowded mall.

People often use not having a special place or specific area as an excuse to NOT meditate. If we continually wait for the right circumstances to meditate, we'll never meditate.

I give people a meditation assignment: to meditate in a public place! They can walk through the wall and notice people and places, while observing their breath or noticing the aliveness in their feet.

4: Falling Asleep

The fourth most common obstacle to meditation is falling asleep. And yet many meditation CD's say that it's okay if you fall asleep because you are still receiving the benefits of meditation...

The only benefit you're receiving is a peaceful sleep! And yet, that is a benefit too! Meditation is awareness. It's being fully present in the moment. When you're asleep, you're asleep, not meditating.

Here are some tips if you fall asleep while meditating:

Don't meditate at night before bed. So often many of us want to meditate daily but don't think about it until we are in bed or getting ready for bed and then we try to meditate. Of course we'll fall asleep.

Try meditating in the morning or mid-day when you are alert.

Meditate in small increments throughout the day. Again, notice your breath for a couple minutes while brushing your teeth or showering.

5: Too many distractions

The fifth most common complaint from people is that there are too many distractions to meditate. Yet distractions don't have to be distractions.

For example, during one of my meditations, my cat Vinnie came up to me and started meowing. He wouldn't stop either. He wanted my attention. Now to most people, this would be a distraction and a reason to stop meditating.

Instead, I opened my eyes, sat down on the floor with him and petted him while noticing my breath. I incorporated my cat into my meditation. Instead of allowing him to become a distraction, he became my meditation!

If you are meditating and a distraction happens. Just notice it. Allow it to be. If it's something that needs your attention, tend to whatever needs to be done, while still observing your breath!

6: Not knowing how to meditate

So many people feel that they don't know how to meditate. We make meditation more complicated than it really is! Again, meditation is about being present in the moment. It's really about finding what works for you!

Again, you can incorporate meditation into your life without taking time out of your schedule. Your life can become a meditation. It is those moments throughout the day that we are fully present in the moment that matter.

CHAPTER 4

Types Of Meditation That Beginners Can Get Started With

Meditation has been scientifically proven to produce significant benefits both for body and spirit in the people who are meditating.

Because of this, more and more people are learning how to meditate to take advantage of this tremendous life skill. As the pace of life increases and the stresses accumulate, meditation offers a refuge from the craziness of the world.

When you meditate, you improve your emotional well-being. This is one of the most well-known benefits of meditation. People who meditate on a regular basis are calmer and happier overall. Meditation has been proven to reduce the intensity of depression and minimizes the effect of anxiety, making it a major mental health tool.

You also improve your physical well-being when you meditate. People who meditate more regularly have lower heart rates and lower blood pressure measurements. Some people have started meditating as a way to reduce or eliminate their blood pressure medication and make themselves healthier.

There are many types of meditation. This variety has come from a long tradition of meditation, stretching back thousands of years. As these traditions grow and develop and come into the modern era, there have been increased variations and alterations to make them more accessible to modern audiences, but the basic system has not changed.

1. **Guided meditation** is one of the easiest forms of meditation around. In this system, there are verbal cues given continuously throughout the entire meditation period. This is especially common in meditation practices designed to produce a specific effect, like meditation for sleep or meditation for stress relief.

2. **Focused breathing** is one of the most popular types of meditation. In this technique, you count your breaths and count a specific number of beats as you breathe in and then count the beats as you breathe out.

This forces you to have a long, steady breathe, which serves several purposes. First, it forces you to direct your focus and minimizes distractions. Second, long regular breaths lower your heart rate and aid relaxation.

3. **Mantras** are a well-known meditation technique. These are things you say--or even think--repeatedly as you meditate. The "om" is, of course, the first thing that everyone thinks of when they hear the word mantra, but there are many more. Anything that keeps you focused on your meditation and free of distractions is a valid mantra.

Many meditators try to focus their attention on specific things. For example, you may try to focus your attention on a part of your body, like your ankle, or you might focus your attention on a specific spot. This is one reason why many people meditate in a place with candles, because gazing at the flame can aid in your focus.

4. Another of the many types of meditation that are available to new meditators is **walking meditation**. In this technique, you walk slowly, focusing entirely on the movement of your body as you take each step forward. By focusing on your steps and your breathing you create a focused mindset that aids your meditation.

Walking meditation doesn't need to be exclusively walking, any form of movement will work. Some people prefer to do their moving meditation with other activities. In that case, regular, rhythmic activities work best. Swimming is one example, as you can focus on each stroke being the same length and speed. Some people also like to combine meditation with yoga.

5. **Mindfulness** practices give you the opportunity to turn every daily action into meditation. When you are mindful with your actions, each moment is an opportunity to find inner peace and stillness.

This is advanced work and is hard for beginners. Some would say it's a struggle for all people, but by allowing your mind to be clear and focusing on each moment for itself, your entire day can be a meditation.

Meditating with a group is popular. Larger cities often have one or even several meditation groups that meet to meditate together.

This can help beginner meditators because they have the support of a group and a regular time to practice, which can help consistency. These groups are often easy to find and meet several times a week to make it easy for people to join them.

Some people prefer types of meditation that are done alone. These people often choose to meditate in their own home and find that meditation is best experienced as a solitary technique. Many people meditate first thing in the morning in order to clear their mind before they face the day ahead.

Meditation can help you relax before bed, so you sleep better. This is a popular time to meditate and bedtime meditation is almost always a solitary pursuit.

By clearing your mind and spirit from the stresses and anxiety of the day you just completed, you can meet the night with a clean slate which will help you go to sleep faster, sleep better and have better dreams.

All these types of meditation can help you as a beginner to

find your emotional center. If you are interested in experimenting with meditation, there are many things you can try. Try all the different kinds of meditation that appeal to you in order to ensure that you find one that suits you best.

For many people, starting with guided meditation is easiest, but you can also experiment with focused breathing, work with mantras, try a walking or moving meditation technique or focus your attention on a candle's flame. No matter what you try, meditation is sure to improve the quality of your life.

CHAPTER 5

Powerful And Proven Meditations For Enlightened Living Full Of Love And Success

Although meditation often is associated with religious disciplines, modern researchers have found that it can be used apart from any religious or philosophical orientation to promote deep relaxation and mental stillness.

What happens during meditation?

University studies have shown that, among other things, heart rate, respiration, and blood pressure drop. Alpha brain waves-the brain waves associated with deep relaxation-increase in intensity and frequency. Blood lactate, a chemical associated with anxiety, has been found to fall rapidly within the first ten minutes of meditation.

That has been my experience too along with the incredible, ongoing experience that meditation practices reconnect us with our Source. It doesn't matter what one calls that Source. Labels are nothing more than labels. Our Source is beyond labels, beyond concepts, beyond definitions, beyond philosophies, and everything else you can think of.

Our Source is a divine experience of bliss and love that we can revel in 24 hours a day. 24 hours a day-while we are playing, working, eating, loving, sleeping, or talking!

Meditation removes everything that prevents us from experiencing this bliss and love that we truly are at all times. Meditation melts away fear, impatience, greed, anger, lust, poverty-all limitations.

Meditation is unique for every person. While there are some classic experiences that can be common to many, meditation brings you the experiences you need to return to Source. There is no fast path. As stated below, meditation requires commitment. Without commitment there is no progress.

Along with commitment, discrimination is very important. This is where decisions to continue or abort a chosen path must be based on research and knowledge, coupled with your own experience.

It is sometimes very easy to run away from something new (like meditation, sungazing, yoga, t'ai chi, new food programs, etc.) because things are uncomfortable in the short term, thereby denying ourselves of the ultimate long term benefits.

Then again, it's definitely not helpful to stick with something just because we don't want to admit to ourselves that we made a mistake in going down a particular path. There is a fine line to walk and we must constantly choose and reevaluate our choices in light of our knowledge and experience.

How many of us are doing things today that we did as children either because we had no choice or the intelligence to make healthy choices? How much of our lives is really ours versus us playing out a scenario that started long ago, before we even knew what we were doing?

How many of us were lucky enough to have parents who knew what they were doing? How many of us are willing to abandon our "habitual daily routines" for a life of freedom and adventure, constantly connected with Source.

Without commitment and discrimination you will stay stuck in a rut you think is normal daily living.

Hint: normal daily living is feeling every cell of your body vibrating with the energy of a thousand suns whenever you want.

Normal daily living is having a quiet, focused mind.

Normal daily living is seeing the life Source pulsating in everything your eyes behold.

Normal daily living is hearing inner music more divine than anything we have created with instruments.

Normal daily living is having loving relationships.

Normal daily is having everything you need and doing that, including work, which makes your heart sing.

Normal daily living in this way is only achieved through meditation.

Meditation is an adventurous voyage into your own sacred heart.

Meditation is a simple, yet profound, way of reclaiming you - mentally, emotionally, physically, and spiritually.

The only purpose of life is to reclaim our Divinity. Everything else is a "background activity". Everything else! Without meditation, you are not living a true life. You are not attaining your full potential no matter how healthy and successful you may seem to be.

The following meditations are ones I have used on a regular basis and can attest to their power used individually, together, or in conjunction with any particular meditation practice you may currently enjoy.

Discover the wonders of your physical body, the intricacies of your invisible mind, the grandeur of your loving heart, the sacredness of your soul, and the bliss of your being.

Sitting Meditation

Choose a clean, quiet place. If in your home, make it somewhere you can sit everyday. The energy of meditation will build in that spot and facilitate your practice each and every day thereafter. If needed to block disturbing noises, use some peaceful music conducive to deep relaxation. Otherwise, sit in silence.

Sit in a chair, preferably with arms for longer periods of meditation, or on the floor in a comfortable, cross legged position. If you need to, put pillows under your knees for support.

You can also sit up against a wall for back support. Sit on a pillow(s) that keeps your hips higher than your knees and supports your back. A Zafou is perfect for this and can be found on many internet sights.

A silk or wool blanket or mat on top of the pillow will help keep the energy of meditation circulating in your body. You can also lie down if you won't fall asleep. Meditation is not about losing consciousness. It's about becoming conscious. If you do fall asleep at first, it's OK. It will be a different sleep.

Sit up straight but not rigid. The energy of mediation follows the spine, from the base upwards to the crown. Join your thumbs and index fingers together in chin mudra. This too keeps the energy of meditation circulating in your body. Rest your palms downward on your legs.

You can also simply rest one palm on top of the other, face up in your lap. Drop your chin a little and relax the back of your neck. Let your lips part ever so slightly, relaxing your tongue and jaw. Mentally scan your body from head to toe and let go of any tension. Just breathe into it.

Imagine the in breath is going into those places that are tight and tense and opening them up and then, the tightness and tension or pain leave on the out breath. You can also imagine that your entire body is hollow. You are simply breathing air into air. There is nothing inside you to be tight or tense.

Then, without controlling your breath, simply observe it. Let it flow in and out at whatever rate is natural. But watch it. Follow it all the way in to that space where it stops for a moment before it flows out and then follow it all the way out to that space where it stops for a moment before it flows back in.

Become very aware of the breath and the spaces between the breaths. Relax deeper and deeper with each breath.

Sometimes it helps to relax and focus the mind by giving it a word or phrase to repeat. Anything of a very high vibration consistent with your beliefs will do.

Repeat the word(s) Ham Sa (the natural sound of the breath which means I am That-Ham as you breathe in and Sa as you breathe out), love, Christ, Jesus, Allah, Om, I Am, Om Namah Shivaya (I honor the God within me), Peace, or whatever is comfortable and meaningful for you.

Repeat it as you breathe in and as you breathe out. Eventually the words will fall away. They are just a tool to relax your mind. When your mind becomes restless again, start repeating the word or phrase you have chosen and let it help still your mind.

Do not give up. Your mind will not become quiet immediately. This is a lifelong practice that is absolutely necessary to a fully functional and blissful life that is not dependent on anything outside yourself to create health, wealth, bliss, and fulfilling your service on earth.

Start with just 5 minutes a day. Add a minute a day until you reach 30 minutes. Then sit for 30 minutes twice a day-once upon arising and once before retiring.

You can even practice whenever you get 5 minutes or so. For instance, meditate when you get somewhere early for an appointment, after meals, or waiting for someone who is late (instead of getting upset). Be creative.

While 5 minutes may seem like 5 hours when you are beginning, 1 or even 2 hours of meditation will eventually go by like 5 minutes and leave you feeling better than ever.

The Inner Smile Meditation

Smiling is miraculous. It takes far less effort and far less facial muscles to smile than to frown or just be without a smile. Don't you feel your whole face light up whenever you smile?

Have you ever seen pictures or been in the presence of saints and fully realized Masters? Their smile is ever present, even when they're not smiling. You can see they have tapped into a realm of happiness, actually a cavern of bliss, deep inside themselves that is always there.

And that inner smile is always there in you too! You just have to know how to access it.

It's one of the great secrets of t'ai chi - focusing on the inner smile in the lower abdomen (the t'an t'ien located about 2 inches below the navel). With practice, you'll be able to focus on this inner smile at any time and thereby instantly change how you mentally, emotionally, and physically are processing specific events in your life that may be temporarily causing you to do something other than smile.

Sit quietly. Take several deep relaxing breaths through your nose. Rub your palms together and create some warmth. Place one palm on each side of your face and start making circles outward with them, massaging your face. Then, consciously relax your forehead, eyebrows, and skin. Imagine an inner smile deep in your abdomen.

Allow this smile to move up through your heart and throat into your face. Let this "happy feeling" smile into your lips, eyes, cheeks, and forehead. This smile will activate the thymus gland which in turn strengthens the immune system. Continue smiling into your body and become aware of more and more parts smiling and smiling.

Keep smiling. The physical act of smiling can reach and dissolve unwanted patterns that have frustrated other forms of therapy, if done with proper focus.

And remember, anything that is keeping you from smiling is not really you. You are laughter. You are love. You are light. You are energy. It's time you experience yourself for who you really are. It's time to wake up and smile!

You may wish to try the Light of Smiles by Paramahansa Yogananda, an affirmation to meditate, dwell on, and practice every day!

"I will light the match of smiles. My gloom veil will disappear. I shall behold my soul in the light of my smiles, hidden behind the accumulated darkness of ages.

When I find myself, I shall race through all hearts with the torch of my soul-smiles. My heart will smile first, then my eyes and my face. Everybody-part will shine in the light of smiles.

I will run amid the thickets of melancholy hearts and make a bonfire of all sorrows. I am the irresistible fire of smiles. I will fan myself with the breeze of God-joy and blaze my way through the darkness of all minds.

My smiles will convey His smiles and whoever meets me will catch a whiff of my divine joy. I will carry fragrant purifying torches of smiles for all hearts."

Nei Gung Meditation

I practiced it every night before going to sleep for many months. After several rounds of repeating the phrases, I would fall asleep and sleep very peacefully.

Then, one night, I decided I wasn't going to simply fall asleep while repeating the phrases. I was going to keep repeating them over and over again, all night if necessary, until something happened-until I had an experience of something other than falling asleep.

I don't remember how many repetitions it took (somewhere between 11 and 20) but at one point, the repetitions stopped and every cell of my body filled with this delicious, vibrating energy.

I could feel this energy vibrating in every cell. It was wonderful. And my sense of hearing was heightened. I could hear sounds that were heretofore inaudible from other parts of the house and outside.

I was in awe and though I tried to hold on to this incredible awareness, I drifted to sleep. And I've never had a problem falling asleep since. Once my head contacts the pillow and I repeat a few times, I'm asleep. Since this night, I've only used this meditation on a few occasions when I've really felt like something was stuck in my life.

Standing Meditation

This means Standing Like A Tree, and some wonderful poetry on the nature of trees which can be used as contemplations while doing this incredible internal exercise. These postures can also be done simultaneously while sungazing (a very dynamic duo!).

Start by doing any combination of these poses for five minutes. I suggest doing one of each as each one has its own unique property. After three weeks, increase this to ten minutes, divided equally among the poses.

Hold them for a total of 15 minutes the next three weeks, 25 minutes the following three weeks, and increase this to 25 minutes thereafter. 25 minutes is enough to refresh your entire system.

At first 30 seconds may seem like lifetimes; five minutes may be torture. The boredom may drive you crazy. These reactions are simply the evidence of the constant tension in your nervous system and proof that you need this meditation/exercise!

Once I attained 25 minutes, I stopped holding these postures for this length of time as an everyday practice. I continue to use the postures at the end of my qigong workouts and in connection with sungazing.

With legs still shoulder width apart, toes forward, knees bent, and weight equal on both legs and equal between the balls and heels of the feet, completely relax-being careful not to extend your knees over your toes. Let your hands hang at your sides, palms toward your legs.

Imagine a string is attached to the top of your spine, in line with the tips of your ears at the top of your skull, effortlessly lifting and supporting. Let the bottom of your spine unfold downward so that neither your belly nor your bottom is sticking out.

The tip of your head (above the tips of your ears), the t'an t'ien (the space about 2 inches below your navel and the power center of your body), and the midpoint of your feet are in line. Your whole frame is suspended from the top of your head. You hang from it like a puppet or a garment on a coat hanger.

From below your kneecaps, your roots extend downward. From your knees upward, you rise like a tree, resting calmly between the earth and the sky. Your eyes look forward and slightly downward. Drop your chin a little so that your throat is not pushed forward. Release any tension in your neck. Relax your hips and belly.

Let the breath be free to flow in and out at its own natural pace. Inhale and exhale gently through your nose only. Your mouth should be closed but not tightly shut. Don't clamp your teeth shut. If saliva forms, swallow it. Relax even more by telling any tight spots in your body that they are relaxed (i.e., "My knees are relaxed. My shoulders are relaxed.").

Imagine you're sitting on a huge balloon that takes your weight behind you, like a beach ball on the sand. There are also balloons behind your knees, totally supporting you. Hold this first position for the desired amount of time. In all the positions, stand as still and motionless as a giant tree on a totally peaceful day.

Holding The Balloon

From the above pose sink down a little more-about two inches. Raise your arms to form an open circle in front of your chest at about shoulder level. Your open palms face your chest, fingers spread. The distance between the fingertips of your hands is the equivalent of one to three fists (3 - 9 inches).

The tops of your thumbs are no higher than your shoulders. Your wrists are as wide apart as your shoulders. Your elbows are slightly lower than your wrists and shoulders. The inner angle between your upper arm and forearm is slightly more than 90 degrees.

Imagine you're holding a large inflated balloon between your hands, forearms, and chest. You are gently keeping it in place without tension. Your armpits and upper arms rest on two small balloons. Your elbows rest on two large balloons that float on the surface of a pond. The weight on your feet shifts slightly forward. Relax into it!

Holding Your Belly

You are now sinking down about 2-4 inches. Drop your arms so your forearms are in front of your abdomen, elbows flexed so arms are rounded, and thumbs about navel high, hands separated at least 6 inches and no more than body width between fingertips, with the fingers of each hand pointing toward the opposite knee.

Fingers are kept separated just enough to allow little imaginary balls to rest between each of your fingers. With soft palms, imagine you are gently holding a large inflated balloon between your hands and your belly or gently supporting an enormous belly that you had developed.

Imagine that a strap runs from your neck to your wrists, supporting them. You hold your belly or the balloon so gently that there is no tension in your wrists or fingers. Your palms are not turned sharply upward. They are loosely angled along the arc of the balloon or belly. The weight on your feet is equally proportioned. Relax into it!

Standing In The Stream

Sink down another 2 inches to a level of about 4-6 inches. Reach your hands out to both sides at waist height, imagining you are standing in a stream, with the current flowing toward you.

Your palms and outstretched fingers rest parallel to the surface of the running stream. Imagine that you are holding two balls, keeping them steady in the flowing water.

Concentrate on holding the balls steady as they try to float away with the current of the running water. Imagine all your weight is sinking down to the soles of your feet. Relax into it!

Holding The Balloon In Front Of Your Face

Raise your arms and turn your hands outward so that the backs of your hands are level with your cheeks. Allow your fingers to soften, curving gently and slightly apart.

Your fingers are roughly at eye level-never higher than your head. Imagine that your wrists are supported by a strap that runs around the back of your neck. Your open hands hold an imaginary, inflated balloon in front of your face.

Press gently outward on the balloon as if to push it away from you, but do not tense your muscles. Imagine you are guiding the balloon away from you. Your weight shifts back a little toward your heels. Relax into it!

Return to the beginning position with hands at the side for about 1 minute.

Moving Meditations

T'ai Chi and various Qigong practices are moving forms of meditation. They are an excellent way to still the mind while in motion; create a strong, flexible, and healthy body; open up the body's various energy channels; and prepare the body for deeper states of sitting meditation.

It is my experience that someone who practices T'ai Chi, Qigong, or Yoga in addition to their other meditation practices, will make faster progress on their path to living in their true state of love and bliss at all times than someone who just meditates. I invite you to find a class with an experienced instructor instead of trying to learn from a video/dvd. You'll be glad you did!

Meditating on the Sun

There are several methods of sun meditation (sungazing), several chat rooms devoted to sungazing, and several websites with related information.

Not all of the information is factual and it behooves anyone who decides to practice this ancient and life transforming technique to become informed by reading as much as they can and by talking with other experienced sungazers.

For an in depth discussion on Meditating on the Sun, please see my chapter with that title.

People who meditate experience better health than others over a wide range of conditions.

Significantly more subjects in the relaxation group reported improved relationships, general health, and enjoyment of life.

Meditation has been shown to contribute to the development of life purpose and satisfaction which reduces depression and anxiety, the psychological end products of the stress response.

Meditation has been shown to have a positive impact on heart rate, blood pressure, oxygen consumption and metabolic activity, distribution of blood flow, muscle tension, and the alleviation of pain.

Meditation helps people observe and identify the characteristic thought patterns with which they respond to outer circumstances. Feelings from the past are often released. As these patterns are explored, people learn that it is possible to develop new ways of responding to outer circumstances.

Meditation brings about a reduction in artery wall thickening, reduced heart rate and blood pressure, decreased respiratory rate and oxygen consumption, increase regularity and amplitude of -EEG activity, reduced blood lactate level and other metabolic effects, along with the subjective experience of peace, relaxation, and contentment, and an increased responsiveness to stressful events with quicker recovery.

While these effects are also characteristic of eyes-closed rest, or sleep, the majority of studies have found these effects to be greater in meditation.

Meditation modifies the depression of cellular immunity associated with stress. Regular meditation has reduced plasma cholesterol and the number of cigarettes smoked.

To really supercharge your meditations and establish an instant and infinite awakening to your Divinity, I highly recommend finding a living Master who can ignite and guide your spiritual awakening to its blissful reunion with God.

CHAPTER 6

How to Choose a Meditation

Mindfulness, Zen, the Transcendental Meditation technique and many other practices have become household words. Hundreds of peer-reviewed scientific research studies have demonstrated the efficacy of meditation for improving health, preventing disease, accelerating personal growth and even reversal of aging.

But with so many different methods of meditation available, how does one choose a suitable, effective meditation technique for oneself or one's family? Here are some timesaving tips from a longtime meditator and 35-year meditation teacher to help you evaluate which meditation might be best for you.

Meditation techniques are not all the same!

The first step is to recognize that not all meditation techniques are the same. The various meditation practices engage the mind in different ways.

Vipassna, also commonly (and perhaps loosely) known as mindfulness meditation, emphasizes dispassionate observation and, in its more philosophical form, the contemplation of impermanence, sometimes focusing on the interconnection between mind and body.

Zen Buddhist practices are likely to use concentration, whether directed at one's breath or at trying to grasp a Zen koan. The Transcendental Meditation technique uses effortless attention to experience subtle states of thought and 'transcend' by use of a specialized mantra.

Christian Centering Prayer uses a word of worship to stimulate receptiveness to God. And this is only a small sampling of the variety of practices commonly lumped together as 'meditation.'

Different techniques have different aims, employ a variety of procedures and naturally produce different results. In determining which technique among this wide variety of practices might best suit your purposes, start by asking yourself what you want out of meditation, and how much time you're willing to give it.

Some meditation programs emphasize regular or twice-daily practice over time to gain maximum benefit and evolve to higher stages of personal growth, while other practices are intended for an occasional inspirational boost or to chill when you're stressed.

Another question to ask yourself: do you want a meditation practice that comes with a religion, philosophy or way of life?

Many practices, such as Buddhist and Taoist practices, are interwoven into a conceptual world view that's an intricate part of the practice-whether it's an approach that contemplates the cosmos and human mind as inseparable elements of a single order, or a world view that strives to get beyond all dogma and see the world as it truly is, it's still another mentally conceived world view.

Other practices, such as the form of mindfulness meditation now popular in the West, or the Transcendental Meditation technique, are secular in nature and can be practiced without embracing any particular philosophy, religion or way of life.

Are you seeking to achieve inspiration and insights during the meditation experience? Meditations that fall into this category are contemplative techniques. They promise greater depth of understanding about the topic being contemplated and help the intellect fathom various avenues of thought.

These types of meditations can be pleasant and emotionally uplifting, especially if there is no straining or mind control involved. Often these practices are performed with the guidance of a CD, instructor or derived from a book.

A scientific approach:

Though proponents of most meditation practices claim health benefits, frequently these claims of benefit cite scientific research that was actually conducted on other forms of meditation, and not on the practice being promoted. Yet research has clearly shown that not all meditations give the same results.

If you're choosing a meditation for a specific health benefit, check the research being used and verify that a particular benefit was actually done on that specific meditation technique and not on some other practice.

While you are looking into the research, be sure the study was peer-reviewed and published in a reputable scientific or academic journal. If a study showing a specific benefit-such as deep relaxation or reduced anxiety-was replicated by several other research studies on that same practice, then the science is more compelling.

When it comes to reducing stress and anxiety, scientists have again found that all meditation practices are not equally effective. Practices that employ concentration have been found to actually increase anxiety, and the same meta-study found that most meditation techniques are no more effective than a placebo at reducing anxiety.

The Transcendental Meditation technique is the only mind/body practice that has been shown both in independent clinical trials and meta-analyses to significantly lower high blood pressure in hypertensive patients.

To determine if a particular form of meditation has scientific evidence supporting a specific benefit, you can do a search at PubMed or through Google's academic search engine, Google Scholar.

There are over a thousand peer-reviewed studies on the various forms of meditation, with the Transcendental Meditation technique and mindfulness meditation being the most extensively researched practices, respectively.

How much time do you have?

Another consideration is how much time it takes to master a particular meditation technique. Some meditation practices require many years to master and to achieve their stated purpose-or even get a glimpse of the goal-while other practices may take only a few months or even a few minutes to produce intended results.

For example, relaxation CDs can have an immediate, soothing effect-it may not be nirvana, but in some cases relaxation is all that's promised. If you don't have the patience to persist in a practice that takes many years to attain success, it makes sense to choose a technique that requires less or no effort.

Along these lines, does the meditation practice you're considering require the ability to concentrate? If you have a hard time focusing for prolonged periods, or suffer from ADHD, you may find it frustrating to attempt a concentration type of meditation.

Remember, scientific findings actually indicate that concentration techniques, though they may improve focus in some cases, can actually increase stress and anxiety.

CHAPTER 7

Steps to Set Up For Successful Meditation

What is the current status of your meditation practice? Is it in the idea stage, waiting to be implemented at the right time? Maybe you know it's something that would be good for you, but haven't yet clicked into doing it as a daily routine?

Or maybe, you've done it at times, but either been frustrated by the results or lost interest? Or perhaps, you love to meditate and would like to gain some insights about how to go even deeper or make it even more effective?

In this chapter, we will explore 4 steps to setup a successful meditation session.

1. Set Up a Meditative Space

Whether it's a spare room, a closet, or a part of your bedroom, define a space that you dedicate to meditation. You can mark this space with a rug, a meditation bench, chair, or cushion.

By meditating in the same space consistently it comes to represent "meditation" to you, and thereby becomes a space that supports you moving into a meditative state. After a period of time, just sitting in this space will relax you.

Another way to enhance the atmosphere of your meditation space is to set up an "altar" that represents what is important to you in your practice and your life.

If the idea of having an altar inspires you, it can take any form that is pleasing and motivating to you. It can include photos, symbols, candles, flowers, offering bowls, statues, quotes, and so on. The basic idea is to put significant items there-ones that put you in the right mindset for meditating and remind you WHY you are taking time to practice.

If you use meditation to support a religious faith, place images or items that represent your faith on your altar. Personally, I have symbols of several different spiritual traditions in my space to represent the Universal Spirituality underlying all faiths and traditions.

I also have family pictures and quotes that remind me of my higher intentions. The most important quality of your altar is that it represents what is important to you.

Once you've meditated in your sacred space for a while and used it to grow your inner skills, you'll be able to take your meditation on the road and do it virtually anytime, anywhere-no matter what is going on around you.

This is when your meditation becomes truly powerful. Yet, even then, you'll probably really appreciate and value those times when you get to meditate in your sacred space.

2. Create a Ritual Around Your Practice

Set a regular time for meditation and create a consistent routine that moves you into your practice.

One way to support regular practice is to make meditation a part of an established routine that you already do. For most people, the best way is to integrate meditation into their morning routine. This encourages you to start your day from a relaxed, present, intentional perspective-and it insures that you meditate before other events in the day get in the way.

Once you've decided on the time you will meditate, plan your day accordingly. If you are meditating first thing, make sure you go to bed early enough that you can comfortably wake up early enough to practice without rushing. Set your alarm to wake you up with plenty of time.

Once you get up, have a routine to move you into your practice. For example, I first massage around my eyes and back of my head while still lying in bed. I then massage the bottoms of my feet with some tennis balls that are at the foot of my bed when I sit up.

I use the toilet, then splash water on my face and massage my scalp. Then, I do some stretches to limber up before I stand in my standing meditation posture. All of this awakens and loosens me up and prepares me for a good practice session.

After standing meditation, I do a seated meditation, then I shake out my whole body, and finish with prayers for my family and the whole planet at my altar.

Having a routine that includes how I wake up, makes the movement into my practice seamless and reliable. Over the years, I have adapted and grown my routine as needs, insights, and new learning have guided me. Yet, the basic idea of having a ritual sequence has made waking up something that I look forward to and moving into my practice easy and natural.

3. Adjust Your Posture

If you search for photos of people meditating, nine times out of ten you'll find them seated in a cross-legged position. Unfortunately, this gives many people the impression that this is the way to meditate. I heartily disagree.

In fact, unless you've grown up in a culture in which that is the way you normally sit, I encourage you to sit on a chair, bench, or bed that puts the soles of your feet flat on the floor and parallel with each other, with your hips level with or slightly above your knees.

Having the soles of your feet flat on the floor and parallel to each other puts you in a "grounded" position that also bio-mechanically aligns your feet, knees, and hips. This position is easy on your joints.

There are many acceptable hand positions for meditation-each with their own purpose. A basic starting position is to place your hands palms-down on your legs. This position is relaxing, while it also supports upright posture and alert attention.

Finer points are "softening" your hands and lowering your shoulders to release tension and having a slight space under your armpits to encourage an open, expansive, spacious feeling in your body.

Next, imagine a string attached to the top of your head, drawing your spine into an upright position. Tuck your chin slightly to lengthen the back of your neck and put a subtle smile on your lips to encourage a calm, accepting, positive attitude.

Lightly close your eyes to support you in focusing inwardly. Unless you are using a technique that focuses on energy above your head, direct your gaze slightly downward. After practicing a while, you may notice that your eyes naturally open just slightly, with a soft focus to the outer environment.

Finally, sit forward on the front edge of your seat. Sit far enough forward so you feel some weight in your feet, which encourages a grounded, present feeling in your body. Sitting without back support also aligns and strengthens your spine, which has an empowering affect.

As you align and strengthen your spine, you are more likely to stay aligned with your higher intentions and feel strong in following them, rather than getting distracted and swayed by less important desires. You develop a strong "backbone."

Now, many people email me saying that this posture is just too hard and painful to maintain.

The reason for that is tension along the spine, weakness, and misalignment. Meditation practice is actually a powerful way to overcome these issues. First it reveals those issues, then it heals those issues.

During your meditation, you become aware of spinal tension, weakness, and misalignment. And, yes, that doesn't feel so good, initially. Yet, if you can accept it and observe it without judgment, without fighting it, over time, you'll notice that the tensions release, the spine adjusts, you come into alignment, and get stronger.

A well-known meditation teacher says that some discomfort when starting to meditate is actually a good thing, because it teaches you to be able to observe discomfort without reacting, judging, or running away from it.

As you calmly sit with discomfort, over time, it resolves and changes for the better. This is a powerful lesson to take with you into any uncomfortable situation in life. Be calmly present, relax and observe things non-judgmentally, then notice resolutions as they arise.

All that being said in favor of sitting upright without back support, you might approach this incrementally. Start by sitting forward for just a minute or two, calmly observe any discomfort until it is just too distracting, then sit back against support for the remainder of your practice.

Gradually increase the amount of time that you sit in an unsupported upright position. After practicing for a period of time, this will actually become a comfortable, relaxed, and empowered way for you to sit.

One caveat is that some people cannot sit this way due to severe physical impairments. If that is the case, you can use back support or even lie down to meditate. If you do that, simply try to keep your spine as straight as possible by imagining that string extending your spine, tuck your chin slightly, adopt a subtle smile, soften your hands, and lightly close your eyes.

4. Adopt the Three Noble Principles-Good in the Beginning, Good in the Middle, Good at the End

"Good in the Beginning" means that when you start a meditation session call to mind your intention, your motivation for practicing. You might want to "relax, to be calm, to let go of stress, to be well, to heal.

But what is suggested here is that the more we can expand our motivation, the more encompassing our motivation, the more meaningful our meditation becomes, the more we will value it, the more likely we are to do it, and the more benefit it will bring."

Consider how your meditation practice will have a positive impact on your day, on your interactions with others, and even on the collective consciousness of "all of us together." What if your practice is making a positive contribution not only to your life, but also to the lives of others, and to all life on Earth?

In the Buddhist tradition, the goal of meditation practice is enlightenment, so that we can use our enlightenment to bring enlightenment to all beings. In the Christian contemplative tradition, meditation leads us into deeper communion with God, so that we bring Divine Love and Light into the world.

In a mind-body view of meditation, we come into a relaxed, expanded, focused state so that we heal our wounds, grow our inner skills, be more effective in anything we do, and more caring and compassionate with others.

What motivates you to meditate?

"Good in the Middle" has to do with your attitude during meditation. The attitude to practice is calm, present, non-judgmental awareness of whatever happens. Recognize whatever comes up, accept it, release it, and return to your focal cues.

"Good in the End" has to do with how you finish your practice. Rather than rushing off into your day, it's important to end intentionally and even to dedicate your practice to someone or something beyond yourself.

From a meditative state you can more easily visualize positive outcomes for yourself, others, and the planet. You are also in a powerful state from which to pray. You can use your meditation to connect to a greater mission in life, such as being a vessel for Spirit to be more present in the world.

As you end your meditation think of how the skills you developed and the state of being you entered can have a greater impact in the larger whole.

When you set up a meditative space, create a ritual around your practice, sit with good posture, and adopt the three noble principles, your meditation practice will become much easier and more enjoyable, significant, and successful.

CHAPTER 8

Equipment For Meditation

When your body craves for relaxation after a long day's hectic work, you either take the option to go into a deep slumber or sit back by resting back on a pillow behind. Although this gives you complete relaxation for the day, the same and old weariness catches you the following day.

So, you need to hunt for such natural body relaxation techniques that can relieve you and at the same time keep you miles from any health complication. Therefore, meditation is the best way out that can perfectly calm down your mind as well as body.

Now, meditation for beginners can be hassle-free provided the techniques are conducted with perfection. The following meditation tips will certainly help the beginners.

There are different meditation techniques for different exercises. In fact, there does not exist any particular way to meditate. If you have problems to meditate in the beginning, simply close your eyes and let your mind relax.

While meditating, you actually need to concentrate and then only you can achieve a complete peace of mind. It's one of the initial and primary steps of meditation for beginners.

No special equipment is needed. All you need is you and a place to sit or lie down. Most meditate sitting up with a good, grounded posture. Lying down is fine, although it is easy to fall asleep this way, and sleeping is not meditating. Deep breathing is not a nap. Not that there's anything wrong with a nap.

You might like a pillow to sit on. Some meditators prefer to sit up straight with a good posture, while others lean against a wall or cushion behind them, and might even meditate in a chair or couch.

Some Buddhists use a flat, cushioned mat, and on that another pillow that is shaped kind of like a chocolate layer cake, maybe 8-10 inches across. Sitting on this cushion, with legs crossed on the mat or in a kneeling position, can feel very stable and comfortable.

Some sit in lotus or half lotus (cross legged with one ankle on the opposite knee for half lotus or both ankles on the opposite knee for full lotus). This is not easy for many, and even those who can sit this way will find that after a few minutes the foot gets uncomfortable or falls asleep.

The main things to achieve in sitting position are comfort, so you are not distracted by discomfort, and good posture. Whatever position allows this, including lying down, is fine.

Candles, incense and music can enhance meditation. If you want music, it is best to listen to something non-melodic, like chimes or bells or random flute and nature sounds. Or nothing. Music with words or melody or rhythm is distracting and should be avoided.

Nature sounds, like the ocean or a stream or rain can be wonderful, especially if you live in an urban area with traffic sounds, sirens, people's music, garbage trucks, etc., because the sounds can help mute the environmental aural clutter.

A great investment is a kitchen timer. You can also use a timer on your smart phone (or even your dumb phone if you don't have a smart one). I use a kitchen timer that I got before smart phones were a thing.

I punch in the amount of time I want to meditate (usually 20 minutes, although I add a minute to allow myself time to settle in), and that's it. Why a timer?

Then you don't need to check the clock. And when you start out, you'll want to check the clock a lot, and when you do, after feeling like you've meditated for a half-hour and look to see it's been under four minutes, you'll see what's so great about a timer.

CHAPTER 9

Frequently Asked Meditation Questions From Beginners

There is no one way to meditate. As preparation for the process, begin by letting go of any expectations you may have. For the first few times, just sit comfortably on the ground, on a pillow, or in a chair, and attempt to quiet your mind.

You will probably have many thoughts swirling through your head; about the laundry, dinner, money, the kids, school, the weekend, etc. Don't struggle and fight against your thoughts. They are perfectly natural.

As they pass through your mind, notice them, accept them, and then gently bring your focus and attention back. You will receive a more detailed explanation in a moment.

The longer you keep up with your meditation (not in one sitting, but over the course of your life), the longer you can quiet your thoughts, calm your mind, and focus.

We now attempt to answer some questions we anticipate from you.

What should I feel like after I've meditated?

Probably you want to know if you're "doing it right". Most beginners feel the same way. It is common to wonder if you are sitting correctly, or breathing correctly, or focusing on the right thing. In the end, none of that matters. If you feel better after meditating, you're probably doing it right.

Is it hard?

It really isn't, as long as you don't have any expectations going in. Don't expect to sit in perfect serenity your first time through. It's perfectly fine if you don't. Meditation is for you, and for you alone. It is unique to you. Let it be whatever it is, just for you.

When you first start meditating, you may struggle to silence all the inner chatter you have going on in your mind from one moment to the next. We all experience this struggle. You are not alone.

The trick is not to fight against it, but just to accept it as part of who you are now, and that you are simply going through a personal transformation. With time, you will learn to calm your mind.

There is nothing you need to do to meditate better. There is no need to try to speed things up. If you meditate every day, that is enough (even if it's only for 10 minutes).

What position should my body be in for meditation?

You can meditate in many ways. You can sit on the floor, on a cushion, or in a chair. You can lie down, or stand up, or even walk around! Some monks actually meditate while walking. Place yourself in absolutely any position you want that is most comfortable for you.

How should I breathe during meditation?

Breathe normally. If you can, breathe using your diaphragm, which means air will reach the very bottom of your lungs. This is known as diaphragmatic breathing. It is a great tool for singers. To know if you're breathing like this, your stomach should push out, and then sink back in.

You are free to breathe however you like, though diaphragmatic breathing in and of itself is very relaxing and healing. It may seem uncomfortable at first, but as your diaphragm increases in strength (it's a muscle), it will become easier.

Those who practice yoga will be very familiar with this form of breathing. Also, if you want to see it in practice, children breathe this way naturally, especially babies.

You can practice breathing using your diaphragm by laying on the ground, placing your hand(s) over your stomach, and trying to push your hand up by breathing deep into your belly.

That will give you a sense for what it feels like, and you can then shift your position as you see fit and try to mimic it. Either way, don't fret if you can't sustain it while meditating. Everything will happen in its own time.

If you yawn during meditation, don't worry. It's perfectly natural. When we do a lot of deep breathing, and enter a relaxed state, the body yawns naturally. Don't fight it or think poorly of your ability to focus.

Should I close my eyes, or keep them open?

Whichever you choose. Keep in mind that the practice does not involve actually falling asleep. You are trying to remain alert and keep your focus and attention. If you are sleeping, you are doing neither (and you might fall over, unless you're lying down).

You can't keep your eyes completely open, usually, because of dust and whatnot, and our eyes naturally get dry. You will need to blink, at the very least. You may wish to keep your eyes closed, because it helps to focus on what's happening inside your body.

What do I do with my hands?

There are different beliefs here, and it is unclear whether any technique is better than another. If you hold to certain beliefs, then holding specific shapes with your hands, or placing them in different positions, will have different effects. You are free to search around at the various possibilities, if you're interested.

The basic approach is to place your forearms or the backs of your hands over your knees (if you're sitting on the floor), palms up, thumb and wring-finger touching.

Another popular position is to sit with your hands in your lap, making an oval shape. The back of your right hand sits in the palm of your left, fingers over fingers, and the two thumbs gently touch each other, forming the oval.

Truthfully, any position will do. Place your hands on your knees if you like. Most prefer to have the hands facing up.

Where should I meditate?

Pick somewhere quiet where you won't be disturbed. Meditation requires prolonged focus, and if your attention is constantly being dragged elsewhere, it will be difficult to carry out until you have more experience. With time, your focus will reach a point where you can meditate anywhere.

When should I practice?

I suggest meditating in the morning, when our mind is fully alert. It will help you to focus, and you'll be less likely to become sleepy. If it doesn't fit your schedule to practice in the morning, then do it in the evening. Meditating has too many benefits to avoid it just because you can't do it at the "ideal" time.

Almost There

Now that you've figured out how your body wants you to sit, and what feels natural to you for your meditation, we outline the basic steps to get you going. It is assumed that you already have a time and a place you're going to meditate that's quiet, where you won't be disturbed.

Set a timer for 10-15 minutes, depending on how long you want to meditate for. You should not meditate for longer than 15 minutes for your first few times. The timer will keep you from being distracted and worrying about the passage of time. Try and have a timer that beeps gently, as you may become more sensitive to noise.

Start your timer, and then get comfortable.

Begin by focusing on your breath. Become aware of how it moves smoothly in and out of your body. Focus on it, and the points where it switches from inhale to exhale. Imagine that your breath is moving in and out of a building, its door opening in both directions and never really closing.

You will notice thoughts pop into your head now and again, perhaps quite often at first. Your mind has a certain ebb and flow to it. Accept it, and accept yourself. Your mind and body both know what they're doing. Acknowledge the thought(s), and then bring your focus back to your breath.

If you like, you may count your breath. Start by counting every inhale and exhale as one count, separately. Try and get to ten. If your mind wanders off, start counting back at one after you've focused back on your breath. When you get to ten, start again at one.

Once you've gotten to ten a few times, try to count each inhale and exhale together as just one count. Again, try to get to ten as described in step 5. If you get to ten many times during step 6, try to focus purely on your breath and your body, and stop counting. Do not worry if this seems impossible. It takes time, and you will definitely get there.

That's it! The more often you meditate, the more quickly you will notice its benefits. You will notice that after a short time, you can easily get to step 7. You'll also notice that you get through the steps faster, as you learn to focus.

You might then expand your practice by focusing on a word or mantra of some sort. Anything you find inspirational or motivational is a great mantra to use. Repeat the mantra silently in your head for the duration of your practice.

The hardest part of meditation is sticking with it. Many people get discouraged because they feel they "can't do it." To those feeling discouraged, let go of your expectations.

Without those expectations, no-one is judging your meditation. It is only for yourself and your own benefit. If you stick to it for few months, you will get there, guaranteed.

CHAPTER 10

Developing Your Weekly Meditation Plan

Meditating without a clear plan or purpose is like going on a safari trip without a map. You will get lost very quickly and you will not achieve what you set out to achieve.

A meditation plan should simply set out how you want to plan your meditation for the week and what you want to focus on during that week but be advised there are few elements you will want to consider.

Meditation is a fantastic tool in helping you address issues within your life and the role of the meditation plan is to help you set down how you are going to plan your week of meditation, what meditation types you will use for the week to get the outcome you are looking for.

For example, the majority of people simply use meditation for relaxation which is absolutely fine but if you want to overcome what is causing the stress then your meditation needs to address the root cause of the stress.

Let us say that your stress is being caused by somebody who is being obnoxious and rude to you at work. The clear objective of your meditation must be for you to develop strategy on how to deal with this person because you cannot physically change the other person you can only work on yourself.

Now to develop your weekly meditation plan .

We should always start off with our Weekly Meditation Plan on a Sunday. I also recommend meditating twice a day, 20 minutes in the morning and at least 20 minutes in the night, preferably 40 minutes. Our meditation plan runs from Sunday to Saturday.

Your Sunday morning meditation session should simply be for the purpose of relaxing. The meditation session should include meditation techniques such as the Stillness Meditation Type, Deep-Breathing Meditation or Numbers Meditation. The session should take no more than 20 minutes and could include meditation music to help you with your meditation.

Your Sunday afternoon meditation session is the start of your reflective meditation sessions on helping to deal with the person who is rude and obnoxious.

The first 5 to 10 minutes should be spent on clearing your mind and working to get calm. The next ten minutes should encompass reflecting on the material you have read. You should also reflect in that time on how you have reacted to that person.

Literally in your mind's eye, look at yourself and the other person, look at how you deal with them, how you expect them to act, try and reflect on using the techniques you learned and how the other person reacted when you used those techniques.

To finish off your Sunday afternoon meditation session spend five minutes relaxing before finishing your meditation session and clear your mind. Do not get caught into stressing out on what might happen in the following day. Expect the Sunday afternoon meditation session to last up to 40 minutes.

If you find that you cannot meditate that long, then do not force yourself but do try to encapsulate all the material covered.

During the week your morning meditation sessions are about preparing you for the day. The key issue here is to not work yourself up before you get to work. The morning meditation sessions should be 20 minutes in length and should focus primarily on stress relief and preparing for a calm day.

Towards the end of the meditation session take a moment to

simply reflect on the key points on how to handle a rude and obnoxious person, by simply bringing the key points to the front of your mind. This is simply a refresher session.

Your afternoon sessions are going to be a very important wind down session from the day's challenges. This session will give you an opportunity to deal with anything that may have happened during the day. The first 5 to 10 minutes should be to focus on relieving any stress or anxiety that has built up during the day.

Then once you have done that part of the meditation it is time to review the day. During your day, how did you cope, how did you deal with the person who is rude and obnoxious, did you over react, what caused you to over act and so forth.

Then once you have identified those issues, reflective meditate on those issues for example, how you could have dealt with those issues better, what you would have preferred your reactions to be etc. To finish this part of the meditation off, simply reflect in your mind the bullet points on how you want to react and deal with this person in the future.

Before completing this session each night make sure that you do five minutes of meditation on de-stressing and bringing the mind to focus.

Friday night is an important night for meditating as you need to use relaxation meditation that night so that the stress from the week before does not ruin your weekend. You will need to do a minimum of 40 minutes of meditation if you have had a difficult week. This whole time should be spent undertaking relaxation meditation.

Saturday morning meditation sessions should be used to review the whole week and to reflect on how you have grown during the week. To review how you dealt with issues at the start of the week compared to the end of the week.

Whether you actually moved forward and addressed some of the issues related to the person being rude. This is also a good time to look and decide if during your reflective meditation if there is any issues you need to research that may help you deal with this person.

On Saturday evenings, I like to recommend to people to take time out from meditating and to go out and enjoy themselves. During the week you have grown and now it's time to simply take a break.

By developing a meditation plan like I outlined above, you are working towards the resolution of an issue and training your mind to deal with certain types of people more effectively.

Meditation planning does not need to be hugely in depth, but having a clear plan on how to meditate will mean that your meditation sessions have more purpose and will help you in achieving the objective you wish. Whilst this meditation plan looked at dealing with an obnoxious person, it could be used to for any purpose you require.

CHAPTER 11

Tips On Meditating For A Healthy Mind And Body

Meditation was originally used for spiritual growth, to become more open to and aware of the holy and the guiding presence of the holy. Today, though, meditation has become a valuable tool even for those people who do not consider themselves religious. It can be a source of peace and quiet in a world that is seriously lacking in both.

It can be used for healing, emotional cleansing and balancing, deepening concentration, unlocking creativity, and finding inner guidance.

When you begin your meditation, put your expectations aside, and don't stress out about the 'right' way to do it. There are many ways to meditate and there are no fixed criterion for determining right meditation.

What works for you is the right method for you. And finding out what works may require some experimentation and adjustments. I list a number different approaches below.

There are, however, a few things to avoid when you start meditating:

Don't try to force something to happen.

Don't over-analyze the meditation

Don't try to make your mind blank or chase thoughts away

Remember, there is no one "right" way to meditate. Just concentrate on the process and find the best way for YOU!

To start meditating, choose a time and a place where you won't be disturbed. That in itself may seem like an insurmountable task. Unless you are a hermit, there are probably people in your life demanding your time and attention.

You may want to tell these people that you will help them find their socks, get the gum out of their hair, listen to their rants about the people at work, or whatever AFTER you've had a few minutes of peace and quiet.

Let them know that this is something that you need to do for yourself but they will also benefit because you will be more relaxed, more energetic, and more loving.

When you are starting out, you only need 10 or 15 minutes for your meditation session. This is plenty of time when you are beginning and it may well be that this is all the time that you feel you can pry out of your busy schedule for yourself. That's fine - it's much better to spend a few minutes a day meditating than to put it off completely.

Over time, you may find your meditation time so beneficial that you want to increase the amount of time you spend in a meditative state. That's completely up to you.

A good goal is to work up to two 20 minute meditation sessions each day. Research has shown that spending this amount of time meditating leads to better health and can help reduce the stresses and strains of daily life.

The process is helped if you can make it a habit to meditate at about the same time each day. Some people find that meditating first thing in the morning works for them.

Other people meditate last thing at night before going to sleep. There is no exact time that is best for everyone. Whatever works for you is good! Just make sure that you practice on a regular basis.

The actual place where you decide to meditate is again up to you.

A few people set aside a room in their house as their meditation room but if you're just starting out, that's probably a bit too extreme. Instead, you may decide to meditate in your bedroom, the lounge, the kitchen or even the garden - wherever you are least likely to be disturbed.

It is, of course, better if you don't try to meditate in the living room while the rest of the family is watching TV. Other than that the exact place where you meditate doesn't matter - it's much more important that you actually start practicing meditation.

If you find that the original place you chose isn't working for you, don't be afraid to change it. The same goes for the time and the method that you chose. The ultimate benefit of meditation far exceeds the precise method of meditation that you use to reach the benefit.

One of the easiest ways to start meditating is to use a guided meditation. This is a CD or MP3 that contains all the instructions you need to achieve a state of meditation. All you need to do is to find somewhere that you won't be disturbed, sit or lie down and play the audio file. Soundstrue.com has many such guided imageries as well as meditation music.

There are many different types of meditation. I still cover some of the more common types below but if none of these suit you, you'll find many more to explore on the internet. Feel free to experiment with some of the different types of meditation explored below until you find one that works well for you.

Centering

Centering is meditation in action. Within you is a space that is always calm and at peace. This space is often referred to as your "calm center".

Being centered means remaining in your calm center amidst the busyness of everyday life. Being centered means not allowing your inner light to be overshadowed by stressful circumstances or negative thoughts and emotions.

When you are centered, you are in a state of clarity, focus, peace, and balance. When you are not centered, you are unclear, unfocused, stressed, and off balance.

A good centering technique will require only minimal attention, allowing you to keep some of your attention on the activity at hand such as washing dishes, folding laundry, or gardening. Be aware, though, that your family may be more tempted to interrupt if they see you doing something.

Just explain to them that you are also meditating and that unless they want to help you do dishes, fold laundry, or garden, they should leave you alone for a few minutes. Here are some quickie centering techniques.

Simple Breath Awareness

While involved in whatever you are doing, bring some attention to your breathing for just a few moments... it needn't be your full attention... just enough to bring you back to your calm center. Breathe naturally, or perhaps just a little more slowly and deeply.

Reclaiming Your Energy

When you are feeling stressed and scattered, take several slow, deep breaths. With each in-breath, imagine you are pulling all of your scattered energy and attention back to your inner self... your calm center.

Letting Go

This centering technique combines breath awareness with the phrase or mantra, "Let go." It is especially helpful when you are tense and/or fixating on a stressful situation or a negative thought or emotion. As you inhale, say (silently or aloud), "Let". As you exhale, say "go"... while letting go of all that is stressing you.

Relaxation Meditation

This remarkably easy and relaxing meditation makes use of a little-known secret about the eyes. Allowing the eyes to rest in a soft downward gaze has an instant, automatic relaxing effect.

Relaxation meditation provides a great deal of stress reduction and can be used as a quick 2 minute relax and refresh break almost anywhere (but not while driving). You will also realize a heightened sense of alertness.

Sit comfortably with your spine reasonably straight.

Allow your eyes to rest comfortably downward, gazing softly, but not focused on anything.

Without closing your eyes completely, let your eyelids drop to a level that feels most comfortable.

Continue gazing downward... the act of gazing is your primary focus (rather than the area at which you are gazing). You may notice your breathing becoming more rhythmic.

It's OK to let your attention drift a bit. If your eyes become very heavy, it's OK to let them close.

If you notice you've come out of your relaxed space, simply bring your attention back to your relaxed downward gaze.

Breathing Meditation

In this meditation, you will be focusing on your breath. This is probably one of the easiest methods of meditation to begin with.

Start by adopting a comfortable position. When you sit to meditate, sit comfortably, with your spine reasonably straight. This allows the spiritual energy to flow freely up the spine, which is an important aspect of meditation. Leaning against a chair back, a wall, headboard, etc. is perfectly all right. If, for physical reasons, you can't sit up, lay flat on your back. Place your hands in any position that is comfortable.

Once you're comfortable, close your eyes.

Start to notice your breathing. We breathe so often that we tend to take breathing for granted. So take the time to notice your breathing.

Notice the air filling your lungs.

Then notice as you breathe out and the air leaves your lungs. Repeat the process of noticing your breath.

As you do this, you'll find thoughts coming up. They might be about family, friends, work or absolutely anything else. That doesn't matter - it's all part of the process and it is perfectly normal to continue to have thoughts whilst you are meditating.

But once these thoughts come up, let them drift out with your next breath. Each time your thoughts drift, bring your mind back to focusing on your breathing.

Universal Mantra Meditation

This meditation comes from an ancient Indian text called the Malini Vijaya Tantra, which dates back about 5000 years. It is a very easy meditation, yet very powerful in its capacity to quiet your mind and connect you with your Essence or Inner Spirit.

This meditation uses a mantra as your object of focus. A mantra is a word or phrase that has the power to catalyze a shift into deeper, more peaceful states of awareness.

The mantra most use for this meditation is: Aum. Aum does not have a literal translation. Rather, it is the essential vibration of the universe. If you were to tune into the actual sound of the cosmos, the perpetual sound of Aummm is what you would hear.

Although this mantra is sometimes chanted aloud, in this meditation, you will be repeating the mantra mentally... silently.

Before we get to the actual steps, there are a few important points to be aware of:

One of the keys to this meditation is repeating the mantra gently or faintly in your mind.

The power of this technique comes from letting go and allowing your attention to dive into the deeper realms of awareness. Therefore, even though you will be focusing on the mantra, staying focused on the mantra is not the aim of this meditation.

Trying too hard to stay focused would keep your attention from descending into the deeper realms. Instead, you will be repeating the mantra with "minimal effort", and giving your mind the space to wander a bit. Resist the temptation to make something happen, and allow the mantra to do the work.

This meditation easily produces a shift into deeper, more peaceful states of awareness. (The degree of this will vary from session to session.) It increases the flow of energy to the brain and clears away a good deal of physical and emotional toxins.

Because of this detoxification, it is best to keep this meditation to 10 or 15 minutes a day when first beginning. After a month or so, it can be increased to 20 minutes, but that should be the maximum for anyone who does not have quite a few years of meditation experience. Also, it is advisable to drink a lot of pure water.

Finally, mantra meditation accelerates spiritual growth as you achieve a state of relaxation and self-awareness.

Sit comfortably, with your eyes closed and your spine reasonably straight.

Begin repeating the mantra gently in your mind.

Repeat the mantra at whatever tempo feels most natural. There is no need to synchronize the mantra with your breathing, but if this occurs naturally, it's ok.

Allow the mantra to arise more faintly in your mind... repeating it with minimal effort.

Continue repeating the mantra faintly, and allow for whatever happens.

If at any time, you feel that you are slipping into a sleep-like or dream-like state, allow it to happen.

If and when you notice that your attention has drifted completely off the mantra, gently begin repeating it again, and continue with minimal effort.

After 10 or 15 minutes, stop repeating the mantra, and come out of your meditation slowly.

After any meditation technique, allow yourself a moment to savor the sense of floating and calm that surrounds you. Take a deep breath, gird your loins (figuratively), and venture forth into your daily rounds with renewed energy and a deep sense of peace.

CHAPTER 12

My Own Meditation Journey

There is a common misconception, that meditation was a rather mystical practice that took over your body and mind somehow, that it was something to be feared almost and it was only really practiced by monks and mystics. I couldn't have been more wrong!

Meditation is merely the gateway to the soul, the vehicle to carry you deeper into yourself and a practice that opens up a part of you that has always existed, but that you never realized was there; your true self and that which gives you the true meaning of your existence and interconnectedness to the universe and everyone and everything else in it.

Without meditation I would not be the happy and fulfilled person I am today. It has enabled me to discover more about myself, to realize my true potential on many levels but, most importantly, uncovered the pot of gold at the end of the rainbow, that which people seek and often feel they never find.

It is the complete and perfect oneness; the knowledge that we are all one, part of the whole that is the universe and beyond, that which is nothing but that which is everything. Try to understand it and it is gone.

The beauty of this realization brings many things; inner peace, inner calm and tranquility, profound clarity and a deep sense of belonging, of purpose and of true joy. That is the essence of life, the true meaning of life.

I think the reason so many people never find this or discover this is because they are looking for something external. They seek happiness and fulfillment through materialism, relationships, jobs, holidays, money and so on.

They miss what is already there, already perfect just as it is, right in front of them, and only by letting go and completely surrendering to it do you become it. This is what the Buddha meant when he said by the absence of grasping one is set free.

I have not reached my full potential because that would mean there is a boundary to my potential. My potential is infinite and so I enjoy the flow of life and trust completely in the direction that takes.

Sure, I make intentions and create what I would like to bring into my life but I also trust that everything that comes into it is somehow part of my journey, my life lessons, and so I am always learning from it.

I am a student and I am a teacher. I am many things but foremost I am just me and I am also you, the universe and everything in it. My purpose is to help others achieve their own self-realization and start their own journey. The journey begins beyond the doorway that leads to your soul; your true self and meditation is the key to unlocking that door.

My daily meditation practice, which is usually for an hour each morning, is like recharging my whole system. It's like returning home to the place where I came from.

It's allowing me to completely let go of the dualistic reality we live in and enter a world that you cannot see or touch but that through your heart you know is always there whenever you should wish to be there.

It energizes, cleanses and revitalizes your mind and body from the inside out. It is like diving within yourself and becoming one that is simply nonexistence, nothingness, but yet that which is everything and everywhere. This is the real meaning of finding heaven on earth.

The immersion of self in the silence gives great power and energy, recharging the whole system on all levels; spiritual, emotional and physical. Let it be, without trying to understand it or analyze it or name it.

It is simply as it is, and cannot be found, cannot be named and cannot be understood. It is everything and when you are in silence, immersed within yourself, you are there, you are everything and it is you.

CONCLUSION

The stress rate among the individuals have been found to be increasing with a significant pace in recent times. The tension from which people suffer may be personal or professional, but it poses similar health risks to the body. Even a little bit of tension affects the health condition of a particular person to a great extent.

To help people get rid of this tension and other negative effects that it poses on an individual's body, multiple techniques of meditation for beginners can be adopted.

Meditation is a technique that has been proved to be very efficient in helping the individuals reduce their stress to a great extent. The increase in the stress level of the people is the main cause that leads to the emergence of several diseases. Heart diseases are the most common ones among other health diseases.

Being in tension hampers one health conditions adversely along with posing negative threat to the concentration power of the individuals, increased anxiety and anger.

Meditation for beginners enable the individuals know the nitty-gritty of the meditation techniques, implementing and adopting which will automatically make the process more and more effectual.

In spite of the proven fact that the meditation process is efficacious for all, several individuals are there who do not really experience any positive change even if they meditate for a long time. This does not signify that the meditation process might be ineffective, instead, it means that the users themselves are irregular in their approach.

Improper use of the meditation techniques is the main reason that makes the entire process ineffective for the beginners. Thus, the proper techniques to be adopted for meditation for beginners should be gone through properly in order to ensure that the process is effectual.

Irregularity in meditation is always the reason for the ineffectiveness of the process. Thus, the first tip for on meditation for beginners is to be regular and make it a formal practice. Schedule it twice daily and make it a routine so that you might not miss even any one of the sessions.

Being irregular, will surely not give you the expected result. Going through the proper meditation techniques will help you know the effective procedures that could yield better results.

As per the meditation for beginners tips, starting the process with a deep breath is helpful. This is because it slows down the heart rate, helps the muscles to relax, enables you to focus the mind, which makes it a perfect start for the individuals.

Following the guidelines for meditation for beginners in this guide will let you know how to technically manage the overall process. Meditating early in the morning will serve the purpose best.

Make sure that when you meditate, no one disturbs you during the process as it will affect your concentration negatively. While you are in deep meditating phase, try to feel your body parts.

Doing everything likewise will help you relax along with enabling you to increase your concentration ability, decrease anxiety and anger. Listening to the meditation CDs, however, is also very effective in settling your focus to one area, which is the one-line description of what actually meditation is.

***** Bonus *****

Wouldn't it be nice to know when my books go on FREE promotion?

Well now is your chance.

100% FREE

Click Here For Instant Access!

Simply as a "Than you" for downloading this book, I would like to give you full access to an exclusive service that will email you notifications when my Kindle books go on Free Promotion. If you are someone who is interested in saving a ton of money, then simple click the link for FREE access.

****

Made in the USA
San Bernardino, CA
07 November 2019